Solving the Mystery

The Key to Rapid Recoveries for Most Low Back and Neck Pain

Solving the Mystery

The Key to Rapid Recoveries for Most Low Back and Neck Pain

By

Ronald Donelson, MD, MS

SelfCare First, LLC
Hanover, New Hampshire

Ronald Donelson, MD, MS is an orthopedic surgeon and specialist in non-operative spine care. He has published numerous research studies focused on the assessment, classification and non-operative treatment of back and neck pain. He is Founder and President of SelfCare First, a consulting, publishing, and low back pain disease management company and is the author of *Rapidly Reversible Low Back Pain: An Evidence-Based Pathway to Widespread Recoveries and Savings*, available at www.selfcarefirst.com

SelfCare First provides education and consulting for patients, clinicians, employers and health plans regarding effective assessment and self-treatment methods that empower individuals to bring about their own recovery from a wide range of musculoskeletal disorders. Visit www.selfcarefirst.com.

Please see the important instructions on the next page.

Illustrations by William Scavone: www.kestrelstudio.com
Book design by Charles King: www.ckmm.com

This book is available at special quantity discounts for patient education by physicians, large employers, and health plans. For more information, email the publisher, SelfCare First, LLC at info@selfcarefirst.com: Attention Special Sales

ISBN 978-0-9790387-1-6

Intention and Limitations

The information in this book is intended to help you learn about back and neck pain conditions so you can be an active participant and more effective in your recovery. It is not intended to provide a diagnosis of your condition, medical advice, or recommend any specific treatment.

Not all options described or discussed may be appropriate for your specific situation. You should talk with your doctor about how the information presented here relates to your specific condition. Your doctor is your final authority in how to address your specific condition.

If you have questions about whether a particular treatment is covered by your health plan, please consult your health plan or your provider.

For information on book updates, visit www.selfcarefirst.com or email to info@selfcarefirst.com. Please refer to this specific book when writing.

SelfCare First, LLC (www.selfcarefirst.com) seeks to promote effective assessment and self-treatment methods to enable and empower individuals to bring about their own recovery from a wide range of musculoskeletal disorders.

Contents

Solving the Mystery

The Key to Rapid Recoveries for Most Low Back and Neck Pain

Introduction

A mystery is something that is difficult to explain or understand; a problem in need of a solution. To solve it, detectives search for clues they hope will unlock the truth. Deductive reasoning (if A and B are true, then C must be true) helps interpret and link clues together that will lead to a conclusion that solves the mystery.

One of the great unsolved mysteries in health care has been the cause of most back and neck pain. Consequently, a great many *theories* about that cause are offered by health care professionals. Theories are often portrayed as *fact*.

However, after reviewing the entire body of research on low back pain, one panel of experts concluded that the diagnosis given for the cause of low back pain was "the fundamental source of error" that "introduces inaccuracies which are then further confounded with each succeeding step in care."[73] In other words, an inaccurate diagnosis is common and, since the diagnosis determines treatment options, an incorrect diagnosis my result in prescribing the wrong treatment which will likely be ineffective. It is this inability to identify the cause of most back and neck pain that is no doubt the biggest contributor to the $80–100 billion estimated annual U.S. cost of care and disability for these disorders.[50,51]

When you recover, it is common and understandable to assume that both your diagnosis and treatment were correct. However, since a great deal of back and neck pain recovers, regardless how it's treated, it is commonly stated that it is a mistake to assume the treatment was effective just because you recovered.

Over the past three decades, most spine care practitioners and clinical researchers have predominately focused on finding *the best treatment* for the symptom of back or neck pain. By doing so, they've overlooked some very important clues that could help solve the mystery of what is causing most back and neck pain.

Some even hold the view that this mystery is unsolvable. They think that if all the research that's been done, plus all of today's advanced technology, hasn't found the cause, we're not going to find one. Many leading experts are therefore not even looking for clues about the cause, which causes them to miss important clues when they do come to light.

The challenge then is to determine something about the cause of each individual's painful problem in order to figure out which treatment will bring the greatest benefit to each individual.

This book is divided into two parts. Part 1 (Chapters 1–9) examines how back and neck pain are currently viewed and treated as a consequence of this unsolved mystery. Part 2 (Chapters 10–22) discusses the consequences of two important clinical clues that have emerged over the past 30 years. Those clues reveal that most people with back and neck pain have a condition that is *rapidly reversible*. Unfortunately, even though these rapid recoveries have been well documented as commonplace, these clues remain unfamiliar and unappreciated by the majority of professionals who treat back and neck pain.

This book talks about back and neck pain as though they are the same or very similar problem. Indeed, there are far more similarities between them than differences and those similarities are especially strong relative to the topics addressed in this book. Therefore, except where designated, these two conditions can be discussed together.

You are likely reading this book because you are seeking a solution to your own back or neck pain. Your comfort and quality of life are simply not what you'd like. You are certainly not alone. It is estimated that 80% of the adult population will have significant back pain at some point during their lifetime.[4,36]

For most of you, this book will be very helpful. And because it is very likely to be helpful to others you know, consider sharing a copy with them, as well as with your doctor, physical therapist, chiropractor, or anyone else from whom you have sought help for your pain.

Solving the back and neck pain mystery should be of considerable interest to health insurance plans and large employers as well. They are desperately trying to lower their high costs of care and disability from back and neck pain disorders amongst their members and employees. Some researchers will also find this book useful in guiding their own investigations into solving greater details about the mysteries of back and neck pain.

Finally, this book has been written to spread the good news that there are inexpensive and rapid solutions for most with back and neck pain. The hope is that you will be one of those people.

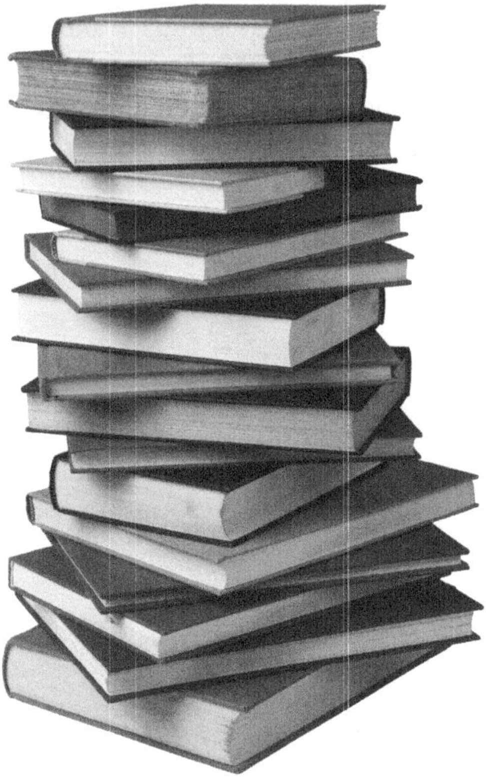

Chapter 1

Another book on low back and neck pain?

There are hundreds of books written to help those struggling with back and neck pain. Most focus on some specific type of treatment with little or no explanation provided for who should, or should not, receive the treatment. Authors typically overlook addressing how to determine what truly causes each individual's back and neck pain, but instead provide their best theory, often as though it were fact. It is as if everyone has the same condition that will respond to the specific treatment recommended by the author.

Likewise, some television infomercials present one-size-fits-all wonder cures for back pain, again assuming everyone has the same type of problem. Often these treatments turn out to be one-size-fits-*none*.

Consider this. If a doctor prescribed the same treatment for one hundred people and only fifty had a good result, we might question how good that treatment is, especially if the treatment was surgery with 50% undergoing a risky operation that provided no help. However, if there was a way to identify which fifty would have that good result and then prescribe that same treatment for just those fifty, there would now be a 100% success rate for that treatment.

Such a dramatic increase in the success rate is not from any improvement in that treatment but simply from doing a better job of evaluating patients to learn more about their painful condition in order to better match them with an effective treatment while avoiding ineffective care.

Unfortunately, doing so with back and neck pain is a real challenge because the true anatomical cause—if there is one—is a mystery 85% of the time.[36] The cause simply cannot be identified using conventional office examination methods or even our most advanced imaging scans. It is this inability to solve the mystery that lies at the heart of why so many end up suffering so much and for so long.

But just as there are different types of chest and abdominal pain, there are now some outstanding clues that there are different types of back and neck pain. There has been considerable research over the past two decades investigating these clues that show that not all back and neck pain have the same cause and each separate cause may have its own specific treatment.

Unfortunately, this information is not widely known despite many studies reporting that *rapid recoveries can be predictably achieved for most with back and neck pain.* But such recoveries require that an individual's type of disorder be identified first. That enables their treatment selection to be based on that problem type.

That is very important news for everyone who suffers from, treats, and pays for back and neck pain care. It is one of the primary reasons for writing this book.

The two questions every back and neck pain sufferer should be asking are:

- How can we find what type of problem I have?
- Is there a treatment that will rapidly correct it?

Good news: it turns out that most conditions that cause back and neck pain are not complicated, especially if the underlying cause can be characterized early and treated correctly. The further good news is that most back and neck pain conditions can be characterized early when they can be very simply and quickly self-corrected by you, the person in pain.

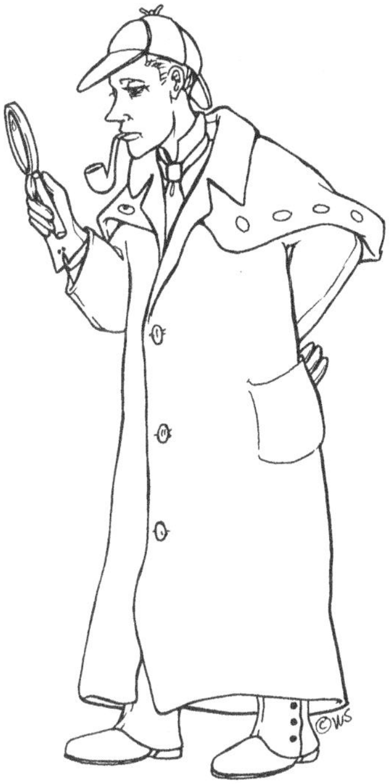

Much of what is in this book will be new to many readers and may even contradict your current understanding about your problem. Some will also be skeptical and that is understandable given the frustrating painful journey you've been on.

But please read on. This information may be very useful in helping you toward a quick recovery.

A detailed review of the scientific evidence that supports the content of this book is presented in another Self-Care First publication (www.selfcarefirst.com) entitled *Rapidly Reversible Low Back Pain: An Evidence-based Pathway to Widespread Recoveries and Cost-Savings.*

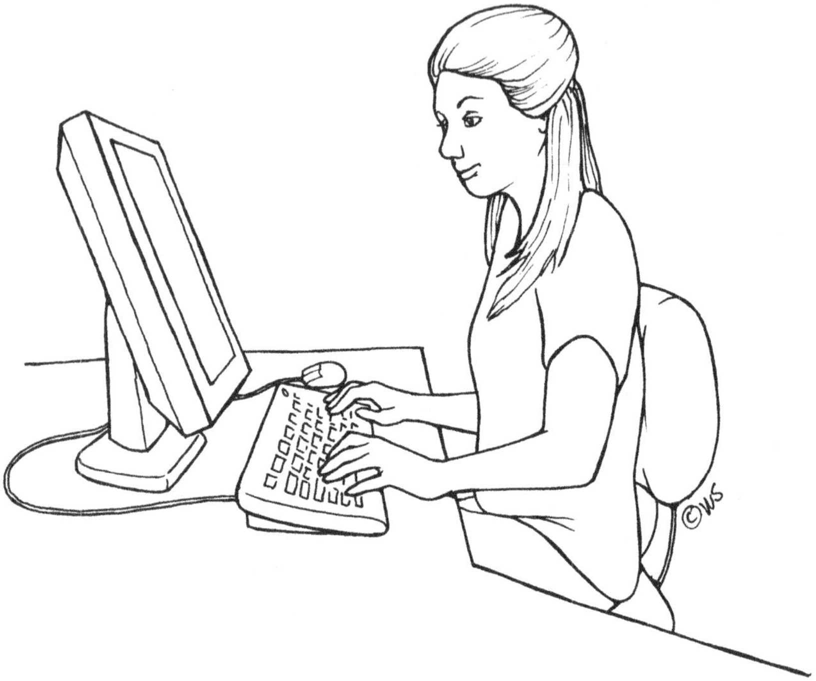
©WS

Chapter 2

Is all back and neck pain alike?

A recent web browser search on "low back pain" yielded more than 37 million sites, and this number increases every day. It takes only a few minutes of reading to realize that these sites contain very conflicting views and theories about the cause of low back pain and how it should be treated. The unsolved mystery of the cause of back and neck pain has led to the circulation of many theories that are then followed by treatment recommendations that target those theories rather than your specific painful condition.

So how do *you* find the best way to recover from your pain?

Knowledge is power: Seven fundamentals

There are at least seven fundamentals everyone with back or neck pain should know and understand.

► First: your pain is only a symptom. It is neither a diagnosis nor a disease. It has a cause and learning something about that cause is essential to solving that problem causing your pain.

► Second: not all back or neck pain is alike. Just as there are different types of chest or abdominal pain, there are different types and causes for back and neck pain.

► Third: the conventional methods of evaluation are unable to identify either the cause or type of 85% of back and neck pain.[36] Clinicians consequently can only offer patients their best theories about what causes it and then target those theories with their treatments.

► Fourth: there are as many treatments recommended as there are theories about the cause. Some theories and treatments are likely worthless. Others may provide benefit to certain patients but are useless or may even be harmful to others. The question is: which patients should receive which treatments?

► Fifth: Many cases of back or neck pain recover on their own without any formal treatment.

► Sixth: Many studies now report that there are ways of identifying different types of back and neck pain that respond well to specific treatments suited to them.

► Seventh: There is one very common type of back and neck pain that is "rapidly reversible," meaning it can be corrected easily and quickly. It also offers very important clues as to the cause of most back and neck pain.

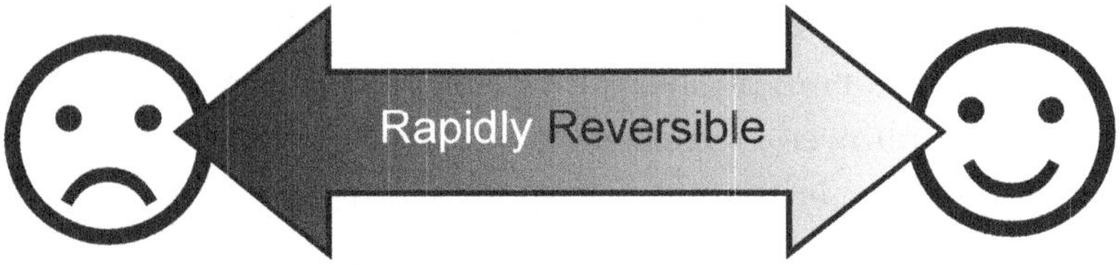

We will discuss these seven points in greater detail throughout the book, but let's first look a little deeper into why back and neck pain is such a big problem.

Chapter 3

Why is back and neck pain such a big problem?

A very common complaint patients with back or neck pain have is that their doctor doesn't provide them with a clear diagnosis or explanation of their pain.[23,79]

That complaint is quite understandable because the conventional examination used by most doctors, along with the best imaging procedures available, are unable to identify the precise cause of most back and neck pain. That does not mean there isn't a cause; it just can't be found in most cases using those methods of evaluation.

Nevertheless, back and neck pain often go away on their own in a few days or weeks, regardless of what treatment you pursue.[21,59,81,82] Therefore, the underlying problem, whatever it is, is somehow often able to recover, even without formal treatment.

Unfortunately, even though it goes away, it often returns a few weeks or months later.[21,59,81,82] Each time it returns, it is referred to as a new "episode." Each episode ends when the pain goes away again for a few more weeks, months, or maybe even years. Unfortunately, it is all too common for back pain to return several times each year and continue to do so for many years.

Many report that, when their pain returns, it's even worse than before.[30,83,84] Perhaps you have had a few episodes. Is your pain now more intense, more disabling, lasting longer than in your early episodes? Has it now spread into your arm or leg and require more care than in the past? Often, after many episodes, your pain finally just doesn't recover again. When it persists for three months or more, it is usually referred to as "chronic." Once symptoms become chronic, the underlying problem is often much more difficult to solve.

Sometimes back or neck pain become so severe that it prevents you from doing things you want and need to do: you can't work, take care of your home and family, or participate in the fun things in life. If you are just not improving, your doctor may offer a referral to another doctor for spinal injections or to a spine surgeon to consider an operation.

Besides being no fun, these procedures are risky. They are not always successful, may make your pain worse, cause new symptoms, and also limit future treatment choices. In most circumstances, these risks are unlikely, but they are certainly possible. Unfortunately, it is not unusual to end up with long-term, even permanent, disabling pain.

But these procedures can also be helpful for many. But who are they? There is no way to figure that out ahead of time. And unfortunately, even those who improve are often still unable to return to their former level of activity or work.

So are there any better solutions? Yes, thankfully, for most there are.

Chapter 4

What is sciatica?

Low back and neck pain sometimes spread to areas away from your spine, meaning away from the center of your body.

Neck pain can spread into your shoulder, shoulder blade, or down your arm, sometimes all the way to your hand and fingers. For those under 55 years old, most doctors agree that pain spreading below the elbow is usually caused by a disc herniation irritating a nerve in your neck that supplies sensation and control over various muscles in your arm and hand. If the nerve irritation is great enough, you will also begin to experience numbness and tingling in your arm and hand as well as some weakness in some of those arm or hand muscles.

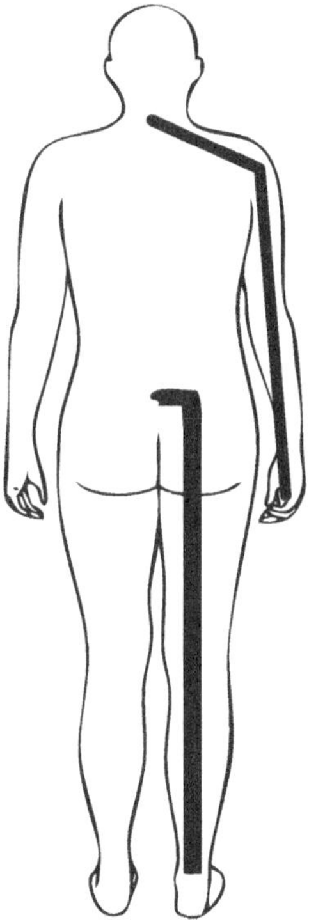

Fig. 4.1: Pain from a neck problem can travel away from the neck, into the shoulder and shoulder blade area, and down the arm all the way to the hand. Pain from the lower back can travel away from the back, into the buttock, and down the leg all the way to the foot. This latter spread of pain is often referred to as "sciatica."

Low back pain can also spread away from the center of your back into your buttock, thigh, and even all the way down your leg to your foot. When your pain spreads below your knee, it is often referred to as "sciatica." As in the neck, if you are under the age of 55, most doctors agree that it is usually caused by a disc herniation (see Chapter 16) irritating a nerve that is part of your sciatic nerve that supplies sensation and muscle control to much of your leg.

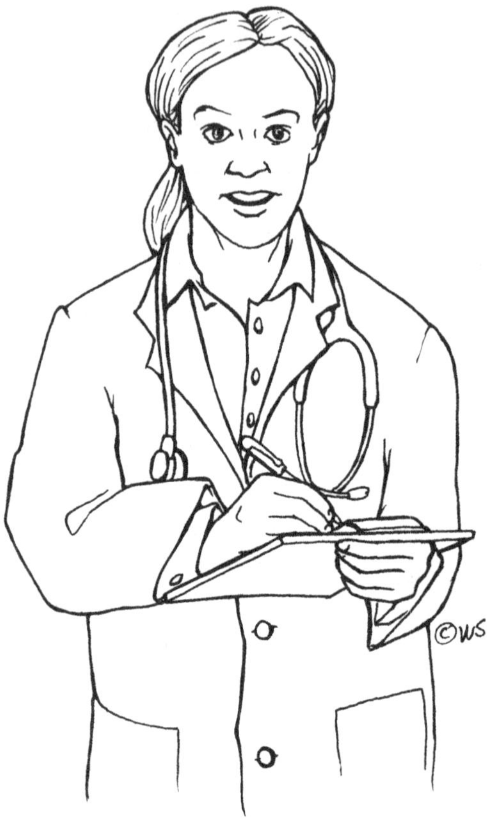
©WS

Chapter 5

When should I definitely see a doctor?

There are certain types of back or neck pain that require special attention. Fortunately, these types usually produce warning signs indicating the importance of contacting your doctor soon for further evaluation.[37,38,69]

Here are some questions to help determine if you should promptly see your doctor because of your back or neck pain. If you check off any of these, contact your doctor and tell the office staff which of these questions applies to you.

Do you:

- ☐ have trouble controlling your bladder or bowel?
- ☐ have numbness, tingling, or weakness in your legs, or pain below your knee?
- ☐ feel sick or have a fever that seems related to your pain?
- ☐ take prednisone or some other corticosteroid medication on a regular basis?
- ☐ have a history of cancer or osteoporosis?
- ☐ have severe back or neck pain even at rest or pain that is keeping you from performing simple activities?
- ☐ still have back or neck pain without improvement after 3–4 weeks or it is worsening?

If none of these apply to you, the information in the remainder of this book could be very important to you.

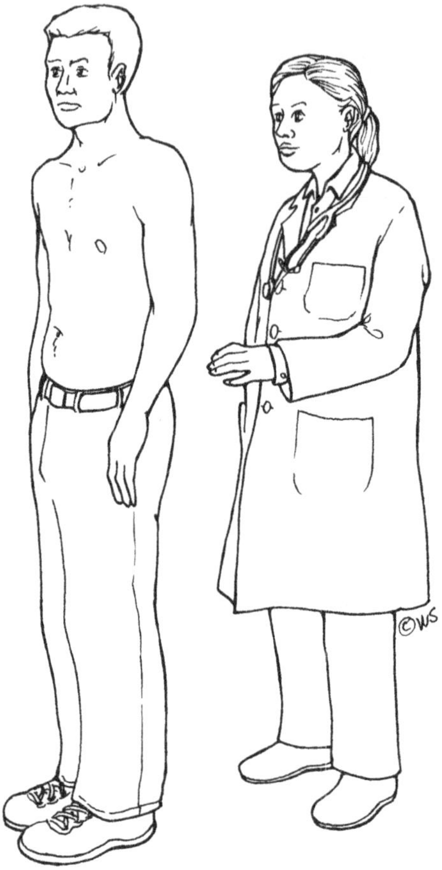
©WS

Chapter 6

What will happen if I see my doctor for my back or neck pain?

When you seek care for your back or neck pain, most doctors want to know what started your pain, how long ago, its current location, its intensity, how is it limiting your activities, and most try to determine if you have any of the warning signs discussed in Chapter 5. These warning signs are sometimes referred to as "red flags,"[37,69] indicating that something more serious may be causing your pain, like an infection, a fracture, cancer, spinal nerve compression, or your pain coming from something other than your spine.

Your doctor will then examine you. While standing, is your spine straight or not? When you bend your back or neck forward and backward, or side-to-side, is your movement limited, is it painful, or both? While sitting or lying down, your nerve function to your arms or legs will be tested, namely your reflexes, muscle strength, skin sensation and, in the case of back pain, any painful limitation in having one leg raised without bending your knee, called "straight-leg-raise testing." Other tests may be added but these represent the core of most physicians' examinations.

This form of examination usually helps identify the most serious problems, which are fortunately rare, including nerve compression from a herniated disc. However, this form of examination provides little information about the cause of the great majority of back and neck pain and therefore provides little, if any, guidance as to the best treatment for most.

Many practitioners will nevertheless provide you with an explanation for your pain, often based on their intuition, personal experience, and educational background. Those explanations are covered more in Chapter 8.

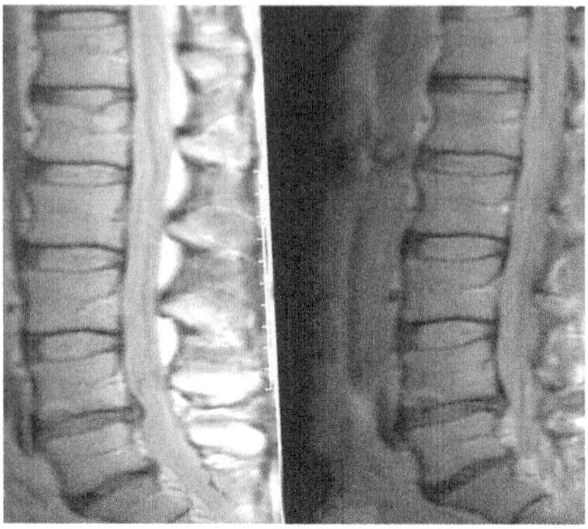

Fig. 7.1: MRI scans are able to distinguish bones, discs, nerves, muscles, ligaments and joint capsules. Unfortunately, many MRIs show abnormalities that are not causing pain so it is difficult in most MRIs to determine what is painful and what is not.

Chapter 7

Shouldn't I just get an x-ray or MRI to see what's wrong?

It is natural to think that our modern and most advanced forms of imaging would be able to show what is wrong inside your back or neck that is causing your pain. In truth, x-rays and advanced imaging, such as MRIs (Magnetic Resonance Imaging) and CAT (Computerized Axial Tomography) scans, are actually quite limited in identifying the underlying cause of most back and neck pain.

X-rays show only the bones in the spine, which do not frequently cause back or neck pain. Consequently, x-rays are not recommended unless a more serious cause of your pain is suspected, like a fracture, spine tumor, infection, or if your pain has simply persisted for 4–6 weeks.[7] Since most back or neck pain recovers in that time period, further investigation is warranted if recovery has not occurred.

It is worth mentioning that some well-meaning chiropractors justify obtaining spinal x-rays at the outset of their care to demonstrate that your spine is "out of alignment." But such "misalignments" on x-ray are quite common in people having no pain. Our spines are typically not perfectly straight and symmetrical, even in individuals having no pain. Further, no one has ever reported taking x-rays before and after chiropractic treatment to show that a so-called misalignment has been corrected when the pain has been relieved.

CT cans are especially good at detecting subtle changes in bone, like small fractures, which are a rare source of back or neck pain. MRIs, on the other hand, have the attractive ability to image "soft tissues" like discs, muscles, the spinal cord, large nerves and blood vessels, ligaments and fluid.

MRIs and CTs are much more expensive than x-rays but,

unfortunately, their greater detail is still unable to detect the source of most back and neck pain. Most are taken with you lying down, which is not when most people experience their greatest pain.

It is especially important to understand that many people experiencing back or neck pain have normal x-rays and MRIs.[88]

Degenerative arthritic changes begin to appear on our MRIs when we're in our 30's. By the age of 50, 50% of us have signs of degenerative arthritis but many have no back or neck pain at all. For most, degenerative arthritis is not painful but merely a sign of aging; a bit like getting gray hair and wrinkles.[9,10,39,78]

To confuse things even more, many individuals with no low back pain also have herniated discs on their MRI.[9,10,39,78]

This all means that you could be having low back or neck pain *and* have a herniated or degenerated disc on your MRI, but it is *not* the source of your pain.

So by themselves, MRIs are typically unable to determine which herniated or degenerated discs are painful and which are not. Consequently, MRIs and CTs are not good screening tests for back and neck pain and should only be ordered in selected cases, most commonly when you are not improving after 4–6 weeks or a herniated disc is strongly suspected as a result of sciatica and a clinical exam showing nerve involvement and neurologic loss in your arm or leg.

Beware that MRI images can even be misleading since a substantial percentage of people having no pain have herniated discs or wear-and-tear (also known as "degenerative") arthritis on their MRIs, especially as we get older. That means that not all herniated discs discovered on an MRI produce pain, nor is all degenerative arthritis painful.

Radiation exposure

Regular x-rays and CT scans (not MRIs) expose the spine to significant doses of radiation that can contribute to the onset of cancer.[71] An unborn fetus can also be harmed by such radiation so these imaging techniques should be avoided during pregnancy.

Patients often push their doctors to have an MRI believing that's where the answer lies. Despite knowing their significant limitations, doctors still order MRIs fairly early in their care, often simply to satisfy their patients that "everything is being done" to identify the cause of their pain.[5] Patients, and even some doctors unfortunately, simply don't realize how often MRIs are not helpful and even misleading if they show something that is unrelated to your pain. Sometimes, for the doctor, it's simply quicker and easier to order an MRI than to explain its significant limitations and even possibly misleading information.

Don't push your doctor for an x-ray or MRI if (s)he does not believe it will help. They're usually right, especially if it's early in your care. Those imaging studies could even complicate your care and delay your recovery if someone incorrectly attributes your pain to some unrelated finding.

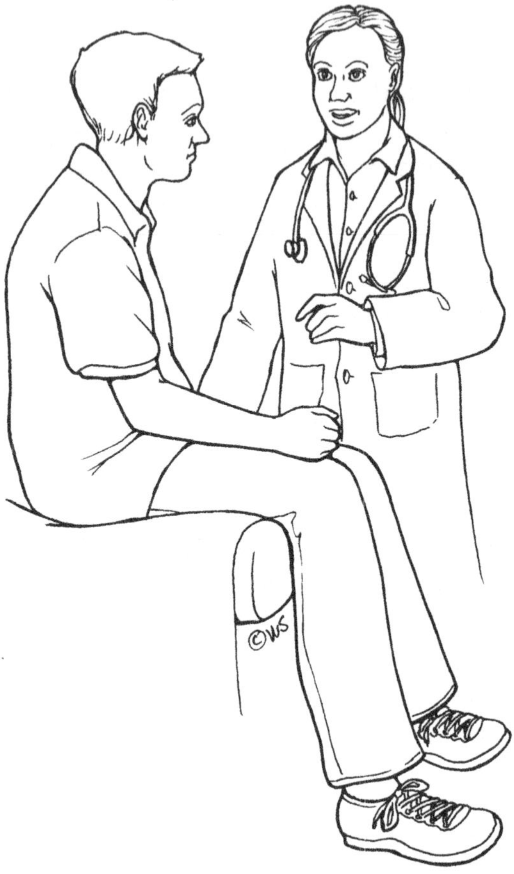
©WS

Chapter 8

My doctor is excellent and told me what was causing my pain.

Once again, the source of most back and neck pain cannot be identified using the clinical examination methods performed by most doctors and even spine care experts. Nor, as you just read in the last chapter, can the cause be identified in most using x-rays, CT, or MRI scans.

Nevertheless, most doctors understand that their patients want to know what's causing their pain and so understandably try to provide their best explanation or diagnosis. That diagnosis could be based simply on their intuition, perhaps on the results of a clinical test like an x-ray or MRI, or even just on a very logical theory that is felt by the doctor to be a very common source of back or neck pain. Some of these explanations and theories are passed down from one generation to the next within each medical specialty without ever being adequately challenged.

To illustrate, consider the hypothetical case where you wanted to obtain several opinions in your community about the cause of your back pain. You have many choices: your trusted family physician, a highly regarded physical therapist, chiropractor, pain specialist, neurologist, physiatrist and, finally, a highly respected spine surgeon. Let's say you see each of them to hear their opinions about your back problem.

After their examinations, unless you have sciatica, you would very likely hear very different explanations for your back pain and very different treatments would be recommended intended to target the "diagnosis" each has given you. Those treatments could vary considerably: mere advice to give it more time and be more active, or exercise with a physical therapist, or chiropractic manipulation, medications, injections or even surgery if a disc problem is suspected by the surgeon.

Obviously, these highly regarded "experts," with their very different explanations and diagnoses, can't all be correct. So you are left with the question: which, if any, of these explanations is accurate in describing the actual cause of my pain?

> Your "official diagnosis" could well be determined more by what office you enter than by what is actually wrong with your back or neck.[16]

Meanwhile, you may actually recover while undergoing one of these treatments. You would naturally assume that both the diagnosis and treatment were correct. It is worth mentioning however that your recovery may have occurred with more than one of these recommended treatments or even if you engaged none of them. It was Voltaire who said: "the art of medicine is to entertain the patient while nature cures the disease."

As stated in Chapter 2, a good deal of back and neck pain recovers even if we don't pursue formal treatment. Unfortunately, even when recovery does occur, we assume our treatment worked but, more importantly, we typically gain little or no insight into how to prevent future episodes.

But of course, the bigger dilemma occurs if your treatment isn't helpful and your pain persists. That may be why you are reading this book.

Chapter 9

How can I gain control of my pain?

Even though most back and neck pain is not serious and recovers on its own, the challenge is determining how best to speed and insure recovery, as well as how to prevent its return. As we discussed in the last chapter, very often, who you see will determine which of the following forms of treatment you are offered to help you gain control over your pain.

Bed rest or no bed rest

Many studies report the benefit of avoiding prolonged bed rest and returning to normal activities as your pain allows.[24,34] This is good advice overall. Getting moving is often very helpful in reducing your pain more quickly and speeding your recovery.[8,42,61,77]

But the pain is sometimes too great to allow much movement and any attempt to move about just increases it. Short-term bed rest can then be helpful and lying on a firm mattress is usually best.

But overall, it's best for most to get up and moving as soon as possible.

Medications

Over-the-counter medications

Over-the-counter pain medications can help you reduce your pain. Acetominophen (Tylenol) is the most widely used. Non-steroidal anti-inflammatory drugs (NSAIDs), available without prescription, can also be helpful: Aspirin, Naproxen sodium (Aleve), or Ibuprofen (Advil or Motrin). Short-term use of these medications is safe but long-term use of non-Aspirin NSAIDs carries the risk of stomach irritation, bleeding, and ulcers. Mixing large amounts of these medicines with alcohol intake can also lead to liver problems and a higher chance of stomach irritation and bleeding. Be sure to follow the written directions and carefully note the precautions on the labels of each medication before deciding whether to take them.

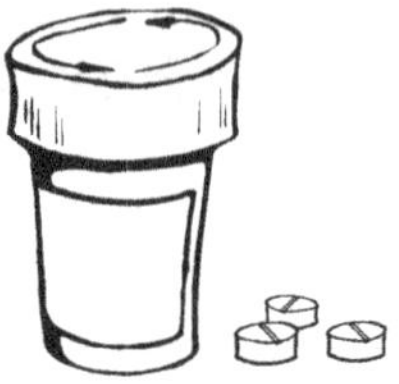

Although a pain medication can reduce your level of pain, it usually does not directly target the underlying problem causing your pain. However, the pain relief may enable you to become more active which, if your activity is not overdone, can be helpful.

Prescription medications

If over-the-counter medications are not providing sufficient relief of your pain, your doctor may prescribe similar medications in stronger dosages that require a prescription. These may include anti-inflammatory medications or narcotics, like codeine or oxycodone (Percocet). Although considered to be stronger pain relievers, narcotics sometimes provide little or no more pain relief than non-prescription medications. They may interfere with sleep or your ability to drive or work, and even cause constipation. Narcotics can also be habit-forming and should therefore only be for short-term use. Someone with a history of chemical addiction should avoid their use altogether.

Increasing your activity level and strength

For those with long-standing back or neck pain that has been unresponsive to prior treatments, perhaps even surgery, there is documented benefit for participating in formal strengthening[48,57] and comprehensive rehabilitation programs[33] aimed primarily at increasing strength, activity level and function with no particular focus on reducing pain intensity. These programs are often lengthy and can be expensive but they also report a reduction in pain intensity that accompanies improvement in functional activities. Long-term benefit may require the continuation of exercises to maintain the progress made during the program.

Other treatments

There are many other commonly used treatments for back and neck pain, including traction, massage, manipulation, acupuncture, and core exercises. Despite being very popular treatments, most have conflicting evidence of their effectiveness and will be discussed later (Chapter 17). These treatments may each be effective in some small subgroup of back or neck pain but are not effective for everyone or even most.

Find the cause of your pain and directly correct it

For most, there is another way to get control of your pain, eliminate it, and then prevent its return. It's directly related to identifying clues that solve the mystery of what is causing your pain. Because it is not yet widely utilized, this option is important enough to the majority with back or neck pain to spend much of the remainder of the book discussing it.

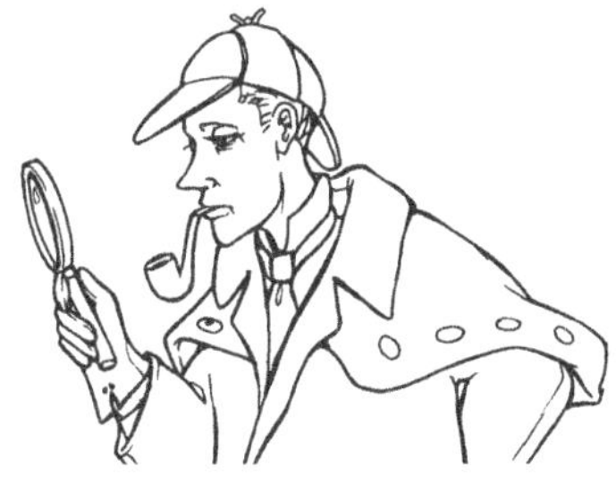

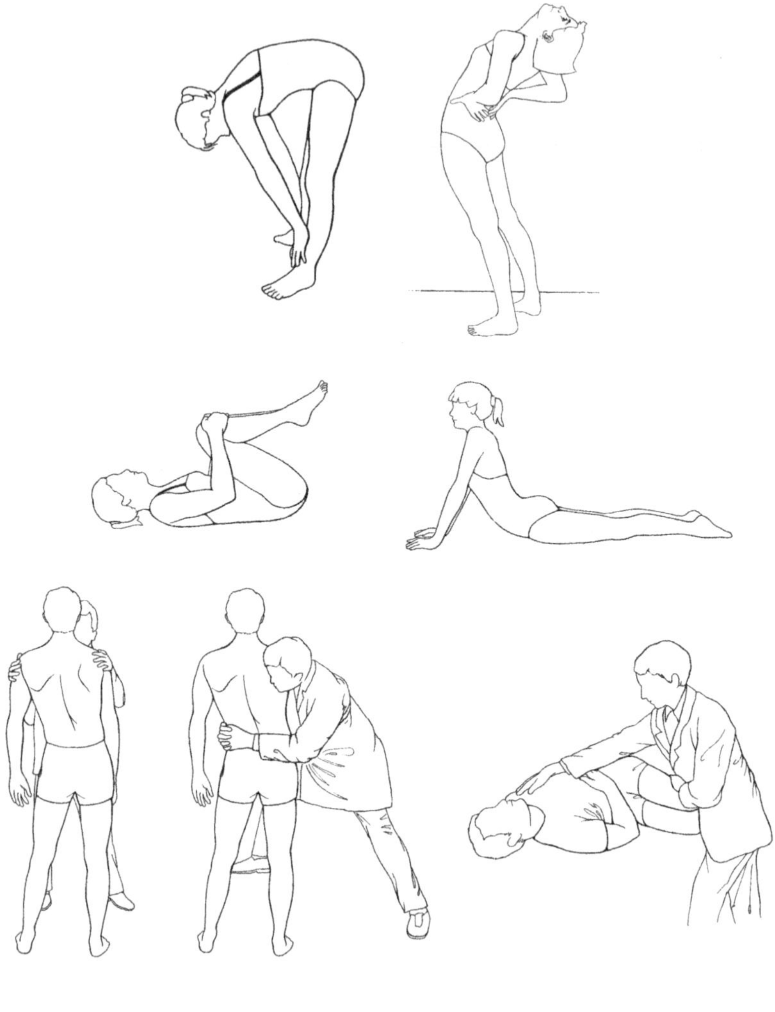

Fig. 10.1: The MDT lower back examination consists of patients performing low back movements in different directions, both standing and lying down, while monitoring the effect of each direction of movement on the intensity and location of the pain.

Chapter 10

Solving the mystery of the cause of your back or neck pain

Because conventional physical examinations and our best imaging methods are inadequate at identifying the cause of most back and neck pain, how to effectively treat these disorders has remained a mystery. However new clinical examination methods have been developed that reveal very important clues about the cause of each individual's pain. Because these clues reveal how most pain-causing problems can be quickly reversed and corrected, they also directly guide treatment selection.

This special form of examination and subsequent treatment methods are known as "Mechanical Diagnosis & Therapy (MDT).[55] Because MDT identifies such useful information about the underlying painful condition,[27,28,86] and because of the substantial body of scientific research documenting the effectiveness of this form of care,[11,13,19,26,43,49,63] it is being utilized by an increasing number of clinicians around the world.

The MDT evaluation provides a huge step forward in solving the mystery of the cause of most back and neck pain largely because it is a "dynamic" examination that monitors changes in pain. It is dynamic by directing individuals to perform a series of very specific *and repeated* back (Fig 10.1) or neck-bending tests (Fig 10.2) while monitoring the effect of those movements on the pain itself, specifically noting changes in its location and intensity. The tests increase, decrease, or do not affect the mechanical stress on your pain-producing condition. The pain typically responds to these tests in very clear patterns that are very informative clues that directly reflect the status and characteristics of the underlying condition. By monitoring these patterns, both pain-producing and pain-relieving mechanical characteristics of the underlying condition can be determined.

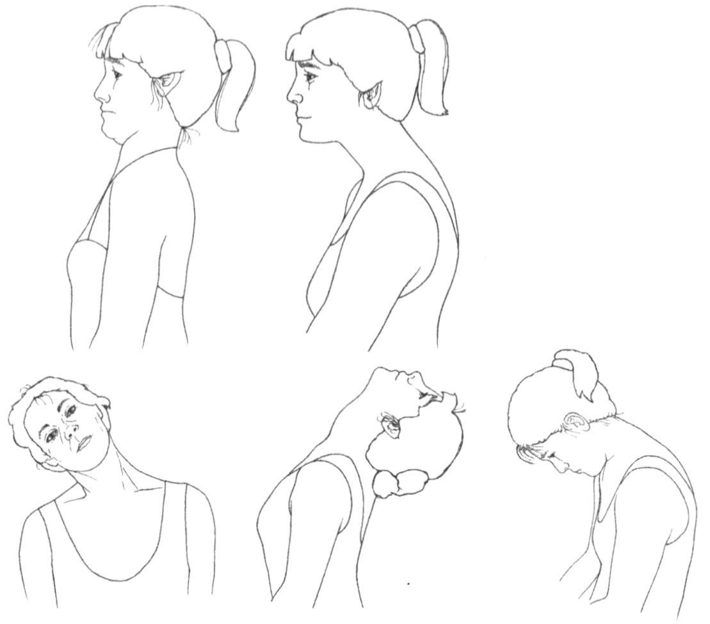

Fig. 10.2: The MDT neck examination consists of patients performing neck movements in different directions, both standing and lying down, while monitoring the effect of each direction of movement on the intensity and location of the pain.

A number of studies document that these MDT examination methods are highly reliable.[15,25,26] Reliable means that different clinicians can perform the same clinical tests identically and draw the same conclusions from the results of the tests. In other words, they will agree that the observed outcome of the tests fit a known pattern that reflects the cause or nature of your underlying painful disorder, suggesting a specific diagnosis. Of course, establishing such high reliability requires that clinicians be well trained in how to conduct the tests and then how to interpret the test results.

Again, this very important information is simply not available using any other method of evaluation, including our most advanced imaging tests like MRIs and CT scans.

Two reliable clues can help determine your type of back or neck disorder

Two very common and informative clues found during this examination are called "directional preference" and pain "centralization."[3,18,29,31,55] Directional preference refers to a single direction of back or neck bending that, if done repeatedly and fully, are often able to reduce and even eliminate your pain. The pain often then remains improved.

Pain centralization is an equally important sign and clue that indicates your pain is improving. It refers to pain moving or retreating back toward the midline or center of your neck or back, typically as a result of performing that single direction of testing that is your directional preference. So pain centralization is the best sign or clue that a back or neck disorder has a directional preference (Figs 10.3 and 10.4).

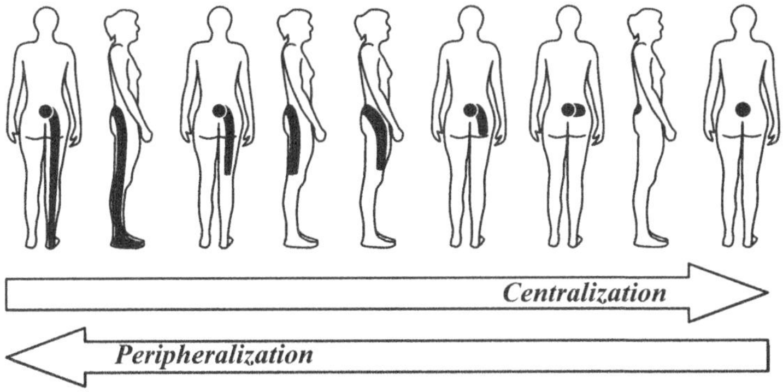

Fig. 10.3 Pain Centralization. Pain coming from the low back that has spread away from the center of the back and toward the periphery (See Fig. 4.1) is said to have "peripheralized." Often, when a patient's directional preference is discovered during an MDT examination, the pain "centralizes" back to or toward the center of the back. This is a sign that the underlying disorder is rapidly reversible.

When back and neck pain conditions have a directional preference, the underlying problem is "rapidly reversible."[27] That means recovery can be quick, if treated properly. This *rapidly reversible* characteristic of the underlying pain source can only be identified and specifically treated by using this dynamic MDT evaluation. Identifying the specific clues of directional preference and pain centralization is a huge step of progress in solving the mystery of the cause of most back and neck pain.

To be clear, not all back and neck pain is *rapidly reversible*, nor is the MDT evaluation always able to identify the cause of the pain or an effective treatment. But, as you will see, *rapidly reversible* pain is so common that there is value in taking a more in-depth look at it.

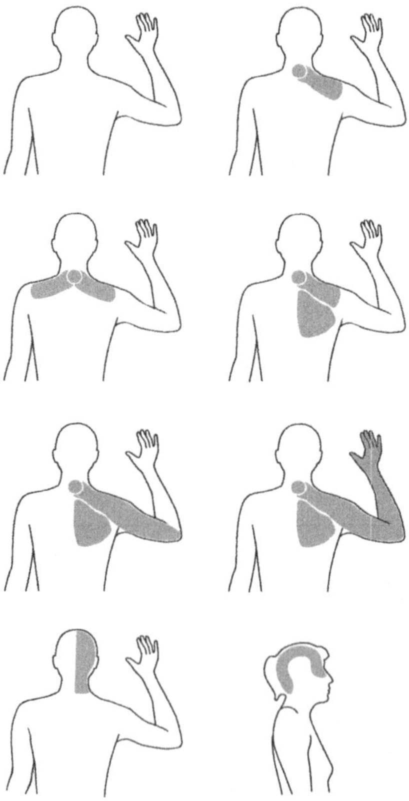

Fig. 10.4: Centralization and peripheralization in the neck.

Chapter 11

What is *rapidly reversible* back and neck pain?

Rapidly reversible means the pain can increase or reduce quickly, and even be eliminated. This characteristic reflects the reversibility or "correctability" of the underlying problem that, in many cases, can happen rapidly.

Even without the MDT examination, most back and neck pain demonstrate a reversible pattern. That means the pain turns on with certain circumstances and turns off with other circumstances. Two common back and neck pain occurrences illustrate this characteristic.

First, as many as 70% of those who recover from a back pain episode will have another episode within the next year.[20,59,81] It's not unusual to have many episodes a year, sometimes year after year. That means all those individuals have an underlying condition that turns on and off, again and again. Their condition, and the pain produced, is therefore reversible.

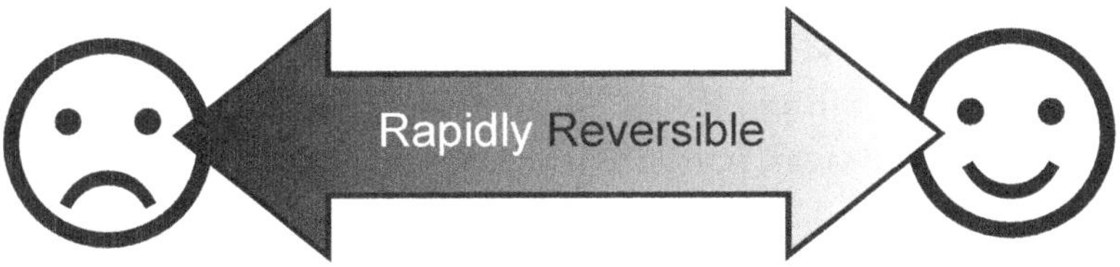

The second example is observed *during* a single episode. The location of pain commonly changes during the course of a day, and does so in certain patterns. So pain in these locations turns on and then turns off during the day.

Specifically, the pain often moves farther away from your back or neck as you perform different positions, movements, and activities: sometimes felt on one side of your back or neck, but other times into your hip or shoulder or even down your leg or arm. Similarly, with other activities performed during the same day, that shoulder, hip, arm, or leg pain turn off and pain is now felt only in your back or neck. Sometimes your back or neck pain might go away as well, so you temporarily feel no pain at all. Some or all of your pain is *intermittent*.

So your pain can turn off completely only to then return again when you repeat aggravating positions and movements.

In other words, your pain and its underlying source, even during an episode, are reversing, back and forth, again and again.

> If your pain is reversible during the routine course of your day, you can be reasonably confident that your underlying problem likely has a directional preference and that your pain will centralize and even abolish during an MDT examination. That means a direction of movement can be identified for you to both intentionally and rapidly turn off your pain as well as prevent its return.

How common is rapidly reversible back and neck pain?

Very common. Multiple studies show that 70–90% of recent onset (acute) back and neck pain and as much as 50% of longstanding (chronic) back and neck pain, is *rapidly reversible*.[11,13,19,26,28,43,49,63] That means that a way of turning it off, often quite quickly, can be found.

Importantly, these differing percentages indicate that, if this type of condition doesn't receive corrective treatment early, a sizable percentage looses its ability to reverse, becoming a much more difficult problem to solve.

Be aware:

► 1. *Rapidly reversible pain is often undiscovered and is commonly subjected to disc surgery.* Since *rapidly reversible* pain routinely recovers if treated properly, many therefore undergo unnecessary surgery because they were never properly examined for directional preference which therefore remained undetected and untreated.

How often does that happen? Four published studies report on those for whom low back disc surgery was being considered who were then, for the first time, finally evaluated using the MDT examination.[28,43,47,60] In two of the studies, 50% reported their pain was promptly reduced or eliminated *during the evaluation itself* and 37% reported the same in the third study. That means those patients could recover nicely without surgery. In the fourth, disc surgeries were cut by 50% once the MDT evaluation was routinely utilized.[60]

Unfortunately, the majority of individuals undergoing back or neck disc surgery are never given the opportunity to be examined in this way.

► 2. *That means that if you have a rapidly reversible disorder causing your back or neck pain, but it remains undiscovered, your disorder may not reverse either on its own or with most forms of treatment.*[28,43,47,60] It often only recovers with specific "reversing" treatments identified during the evaluation. *Rapidly reversible* pain so often persists either because you are never given the opportunity to be properly examined or the examiner is not sufficiently knowledgeable of these specific examination methods resulting in an incomplete examination.

For example, in those four pre-surgery studies just described, many were still found to have a *rapidly reversible* problem when finally properly evaluated. Their problem, of course, had actually been *rapidly reversible* from the very beginning of their episode but, because it had never been discovered, it was never treated properly and so persisted to the point where they almost underwent unnecessary surgery. Consequently, many with a *rapidly reversible* problem suffer unnecessarily, even to the extent of undergoing unnecessary surgery.

One further point: if those individuals with *rapidly reversible* back or neck pain had been evaluated far earlier in their care, they would very likely have recovered much earlier. They could have avoided their lengthy period of pain and limited activities as well as any need for all their other unsuccessful treatments, including medications, lengthy physical therapy or chiropractic care, MRIs and injections.

For employers and health plans, the time and money wasted because of undiscovered and untreated reversible problems is gigantic.

But the question remains: can *your* pain be intentionally reversed? Is it *rapidly reversible?* It very likely is. If so, the remainder of this book is very important for you to read.

Chapter 12

Is my pain *rapidly reversible*?

> *Rapidly reversible* back and neck pain is very common and simply means the underlying problem can be quickly corrected if the right mechanical forces are applied to it. This is perhaps the most important message of this book.

Determining if your back or neck pain is coming from a *rapidly reversible* condition requires this unique MDT form of clinical evaluation. This is the first step in a uniquely informative type of care first described in 1981 by Robin McKenzie, a physical therapist from New Zealand.[52] His significant contribution to our understanding of how to evaluate and treat back and neck pain cannot be over-emphasized.

The MDT examination

This MDT examination is simple and safe.[55] Because there are several varieties of *rapidly reversible* pain, including some with greater complexity that require more than one examination session,[85] the exam needs to be precise and thorough and therefore conducted by a clinician with specific training and credentialing in this form of exam (see Chapter 20).

The primary intent of the examination is to determine the mechanical characteristics of the underlying cause of your pain and, more specifically, whether you have a *rapidly reversible* condition that you can reverse on your own. Without needing to identify your anatomical source of pain, your pain source can nevertheless be directly and intentionally tested and characterized by having you assume positions and perform repeated back or neck bending tests in various directions while closely monitoring how your pain responds.

This assessment and treatment process values many details of your past painful journey and provides the opportunity to partner with your examiner in solving your personal mystery of the cause of your pain and determining how to correct it. It does not go on and on if nothing beneficial is found.

Is your pain rapidly reversible?

Rapidly reversible pain is present in those in whom a directional preference is found. That is the direction of movement that the underlying pain source "prefers" or requires to be quickly corrected and recover.[29,55] When found, the needed direction of mechanical force produces a lasting reduction, centralization, and elimination of the pain as well as a simultaneous return of the full range of back or neck movement.

> To reverse your own problem puts you in control.

If you do have a rapidly reversible back or neck problem

If your pain is found to be *rapidly reversible*, your MDT examiner then becomes your coach, teaching you your very own pain-eliminating and prevention self-care program. This enables you to take your own pain away as your initial step toward your recovery. Until and unless that takes place, you will likely remain either at the mercy of your pain or reliant on your clinician to provide some relief for you.

Since your recovery can occur rapidly, you have no need for imaging or any other treatment, including medications, manipulation, injections, or surgery.

Preventing future episodes

Once you learn how to eliminate your own pain and recover from your current painful episode, you will also have gained significant insight into how to prevent another episode by simply continuing to use whatever movements and positions worked so well during your initial recovery.[76] By monitoring any pain that returns, you can quickly respond and again eliminate it using the same movements and positions that worked so well previously.

Such control enables you to remain out of the health care system and avoid the need to receive formal treatment again and again.

To find a trained MDT clinician near you, see Chapter 20.

Chapter 13

Wouldn't my doctor test me to see if my pain is *rapidly reversible*?

Not all doctors know that most back and neck pain is *rapidly reversible*. Many are also unaware of the strength of the supportive scientific evidence. Even those that do know typically do not choose to invest the considerable amount of time required to learn these methods themselves. Instead, most choose to refer their patients to clinicians (usually physical therapists or chiropractors) who already have the MDT specialized training. These trained clinicians are sometimes referred to as "McKenzie clinicians" because they received their training from the McKenzie Institute.

The unfortunate reality is that many doctors are still unfamiliar with this form of evaluation. If that is true of your doctor, consider sharing a copy of this book to help introduce him or her to the benefits of using these methods.

If your doctor does not offer to refer you to a well-trained MDT clinician, you may request such a referral. Doctors typically honor such requests. Your doctor may not know who in your area is well-trained in MDT methods so you may want to do your own homework ahead of time to identify the most qualified clinician (see Chapter 20).

Chapter 14

Learning how to turn your own pain off

A very attractive feature of *rapidly reversible* back and neck pain is that the one with the pain is typically the best one to apply the beneficial "reversing" force to their spine using simple-but-precise movements and posture modifications. If you brought the pain on yourself, you can also usually turn it off yourself. Most learn how to do this during their initial MDT evaluation. They then confirm the usefulness of these treatment methods again at home and at work when they are able to chase away any pain that tries to return.

All that's required to determine if this treatment is working is to simply monitor how your pain responds to your positions, activities, and treatment movements. It's both convincing and reassuring when the directional movements you've been instructed to perform consistently reduce and eliminate your pain while those positions, activities, or movements you've learned to temporarily avoid consistently cause your pain to return or worsen. That's how *rapidly reversible* pain works.

> It doesn't matter whether your pain is mild or severe, acute or chronic, confined to your back or neck, whether it spreads down your arm to the hand or down your leg to the foot, or even if you have tried several other treatments that didn't help. Your problem could still be *rapidly reversible* if evaluated and treated properly.

By learning the proper mechanical strategies that eliminate your current pain, you acquire the knowledge, skills, and experience to prevent your pain from returning long-term (see Chapter 22).

> The evaluation and treatment of two such patients, one low back and one neck pain, are described in the Appendix of this book.

Chapter 15

What is a "mechanical diagnosis"?

Finding the underlying cause of any symptom is key to correcting the problem and eliminating that symptom. The primary reason back and neck pain have been such a mystery and perplexing problem is that our conventional ways of evaluating these conditions have been unable to make an accurate diagnosis most of the time.

However, multiple studies report that 80–90% of acute back and neck pain is *rapidly reversible.*[31,40,74,85] That means that discovering the cause of pain in that huge subgroup would identify the source of 80–90% of all back and neck pain. That would be a momentous discovery.

But do we need to identify the anatomic pain source, meaning the precise tissue causing the pain, in order to identify effective treatment that achieves a rapid recovery? A very fortunate feature of back and neck pain revealed by these MDT methods is that rapid recoveries do not require the identification of the actual anatomic cause. Simply learning some critically important mechanical characteristics of the cause is enough.

Clearly, if a way is found to rapidly turn off your pain, and it remains turned off, the actual cause, whatever it is, has likely been corrected. If the pain is gone, there is no need to further investigate its actual cause. What that actual anatomic cause of *rapidly reversible* pain might be will be discussed more in the next chapter.

Because your recovery does not require finding the anatomic cause of your pain, the remainder of this and the next chapter may not be of much interest to you. It is included for those who want to know more about why they recover so quickly and easily.

Which theory is the best fit?

Considering the possible causes of *rapidly reversible* pain requires recognition that the pain is not only centralized and even turned off during the MDT evaluation process, it usually remains better after the testing is completed. It's as though the source of the pain, whatever it is, has somehow been changed for the better as the result of performing a single direction of test movements.

Clinical reasoning helps solve the mystery

An important step in solving the mystery of the cause of back or neck pain is to consider the clinical clues about the character of the underlying cause of pain in light of various commonly held explanations for back or neck pain. Again, the two clues that provide exceptional insight into the pain source are "directional preference" and "pain centralization."

Injured ligaments or muscles are thought by many to be common causes of back and neck pain. However, an injured, painful muscle or ligament would not suddenly heal and stop hurting as a direct result of a few minutes of moving the spine in a single direction. Pain from tissue injury would not quickly centralize, disappear, and then remain better. Further, no evidence of such injury or scar tissue repair has ever been reported during the thousands of back and neck surgeries performed every day around the world.

Inflammation is another commonly stated explanation for back and neck pain. This is a cellular and tissue reaction to irritation and injury. Again, inflammation would not quickly go away and stay away as a result of simply bending the spine a few times in one specific direction.

These two commonly suggested theories are not plausible explanations for *rapidly reversible* back or neck pain, nor would many other theories explain these directional preference and rapid recovery characteristics that so many with back and neck pain exhibit when examined for them.

But there is a compelling mechanical explanation.

A mechanical diagnosis: a derangement

You do not have to create some new complex explanation for this most common type of back and neck pain. One particular "mechanical" explanation very nicely fits *rapidly reversible* pain.[28,55,86] Recall that "MDT" stands for Mechanical Diagnosis & Therapy and the MDT examination uses mechanical movements and positioning to test how the underlying pain source responds.

The most plausible explanation for *rapidly reversible* pain is that a mechanical problem has occurred within one of the joints of the spine, specifically that something moved out of place. That displacement would of course be painful and also would interfere with the mechanics and movement of that joint.

Such displacements, often called "derangements," commonly occur in other joints in the body, like the shoulder, hip, elbow etc. A derangement would be considered a "mechanical diagnosis" rather than an anatomic diagnosis. To be an anatomic diagnosis would require identifying the specific tissue that is deranged or out of place.

So a back or neck "derangement" is a very good fit for how *rapidly reversible* back and neck pain behaves and responds, either over the course of your day or during the MDT examination itself.

The amount of painful displacement frequently varies in response to your different positions, movements and activities. When the displacement increases, pain will spread farther away from your back or neck, even into the leg or arm.[56,58,72,75,89]

Also, as displacement increases, the movement of that joint is further limited or obstructed. Alternatively, when the displacement decreases as a result of alternative mechanical forces applied by other positions, movements, and activities, the spread of your pain will decrease (the pain "centralizes") and your ability to move the joint will improve.

When the MDT examination identifies a direction of spinal bending and positioning that reduces the pain and restores movement, that direction of movement likely moves the displaced tissue back toward or to its original location.[62] Successful correction brings immediate, substantial pain relief and a simultaneous return of movement to the joint.[14]

The primary intent of a thorough MDT exam is to identify a directional preference that promptly relieves the pain and restores your spine's ability to comfortably bend again. When found, one can be confident that the underlying condition is *rapidly reversible* with a high likelihood of a rapid recovery.[11,13,19,26,28,43,49,63]

The next chapter will examine the evidence that the anatomic diagnosis for most *rapidly reversible* back and neck pain is a derangement within an intervertebral disc.

Chapter 16

What is the anatomic diagnosis for *rapidly reversible* back pain?

Disc herniations are already familiar derangements of the spine that are visible on MRI scans. The content of a disc has moved backward and has created a bulge or herniation that could be painful.

What are intervertebral discs?

Intervertebral discs are the shock absorbers that lie between the vertebrae in our spine (Fig. 16.1). They are widely regarded as a common source of back or neck pain, especially once the pain spreads down the arm past the elbow or down the leg past the knee. Many also believe that chronic neck or back pain, without any spread, often comes from some disruption inside the disc. But once again, and unfortunately, conventional office examination tests and even our most advanced imaging scans have considerable difficulty confirming the disc as the pain source.

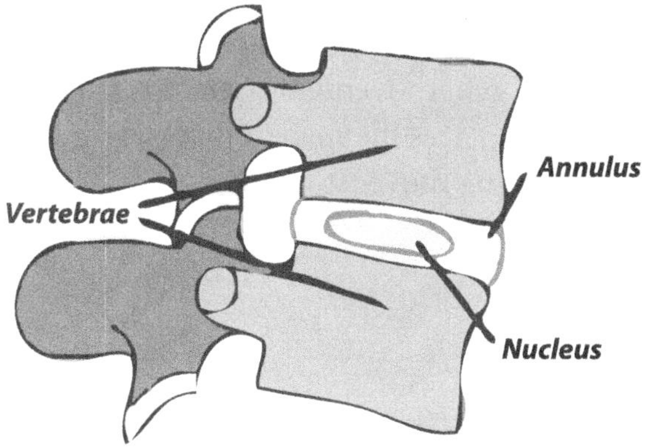

Fig. 16.1: The disc lies between two vertebrae and is made up on an outer shell or container, called the annulus, and a moist gel-like substance inside, called the nucleus.

How do discs work and cause pain?

Each disc has an outer shell, called the annulus, and an inner gel called the nucleus, much like a jelly-filled donut (Fig. 16.1).

When you bend your spine, compression is applied to that side of the disc that squeezes the nucleus in the opposite direction, much like toothpaste moving away from where the tube is squeezed (Fig. 16.2). That movement of the nucleus is both normal and essential for the spine to bend.

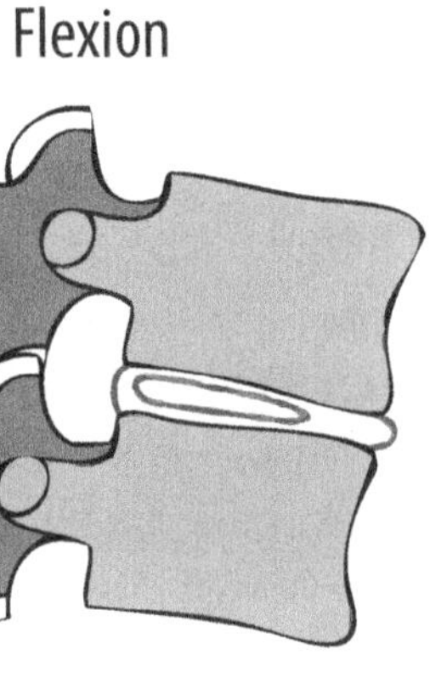

Fig. 16.2: When the normal spine bends forward (flexes), the discs are compressed in the front (on the right) which squeezes each nucleus toward the back (to the left).

If the spine is then bent in the opposite direction, the compression is now applied on the opposite side of the disc. This reverses the direction of movement of the nucleus (Fig. 16.3). So forward bending displaces the nucleus backward within the disc and backward bending moves it forward.[2,32,62,65,67,68]

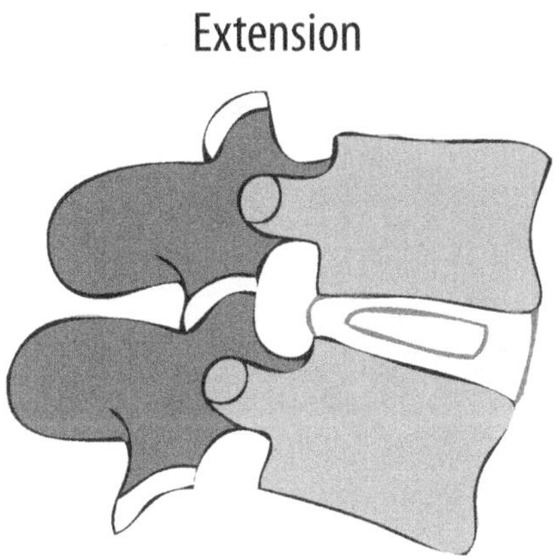

Fig. 16.3: When the normal spine bends backward (extends), the discs are compressed in the back (on the left) which squeezes each nucleus toward the front (to the right).

Pain begins when one direction of bending is performed excessively causing abnormally greater nuclear displacement. This most commonly happens with forward bending, forward compression on the disc of greater force (heavy lifting), more repetitions (shoveling, repeated lifting), or for prolonged time (vacuuming or sitting slouched). The nucleus is squeezed with this excessive force toward the opposite side of the disc which, over the course of time and this excessive force, can result in a localized area of weakness in the annulus.[1]

If that force continues, the annulus further weakens allowing further displacement to occur and the annulus begins to balloon, much like a balloon forming on a tire (Fig 16.5). This is commonly referred to as a bulging disc and can often be seen on a CT or MRI scan.

The pain of these derangements however often begins long before any ballooning is seen on an MRI when nerve endings within the annulus itself complain about the over-stretch and early damage to the annulus.[44,80] As these bending stresses, pressure, and annulus stretching continue, the bulge enlarges and becomes a hernia, meaning it balloons even more (Fig. 16.4).

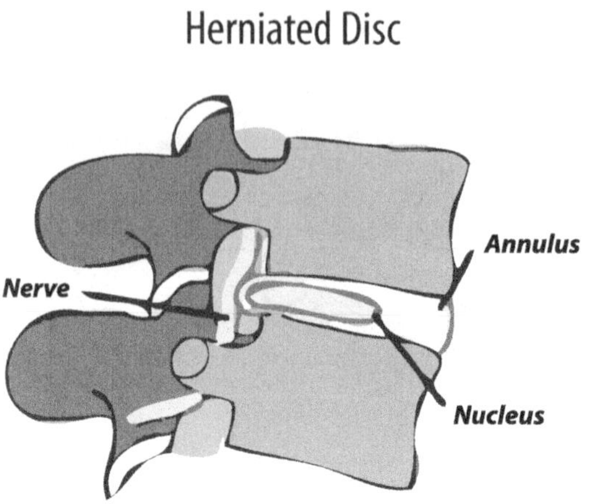

Fig. 16.4: When excessive or vigorous forward bending occurs (slouched sitting, lifting, sneezing, forward bending), the nucleus is squeezed for much longer, or with much greater force, toward the back of the disc. This causes excessive displacement of the nucleus and also damage to the annulus so that a balloon or herniation forms in the back of the disc. Sensitive nerves in the annulus cause pain as does pressure applied by the herniation (balloon) to the nerve outside the disc.

A herniation often enlarges to the point of contacting, compressing, and irritating large nerve roots that live just outside the back of each disc. Irritating a nerve root will cause pain that is felt down the leg, below the knee, and even into the foot. Pain below the knee is referred to as "sciatica" (see Chapter 4).

Although the end result of this displacement process can be an actual disc herniation and nerve root irritation, this only represents a minority of patients. The majority seeks care while in earlier stages of displacement and pain, while the annular wall is still intact and the tissue displacement can still be reversed. This is the group in which 80–90% have been reported to have a directional preference where the displacement can still be corrected.

The extreme of this displacement process finds the annulus ruptured, meaning a complete blow-out or "extrusion" of the nuclear material (Fig. 16.5). Unfortunately, once this happens, no direction of bending can draw the displaced pain-generating nucleus back into the disc. The toothpaste is out of the tube. The

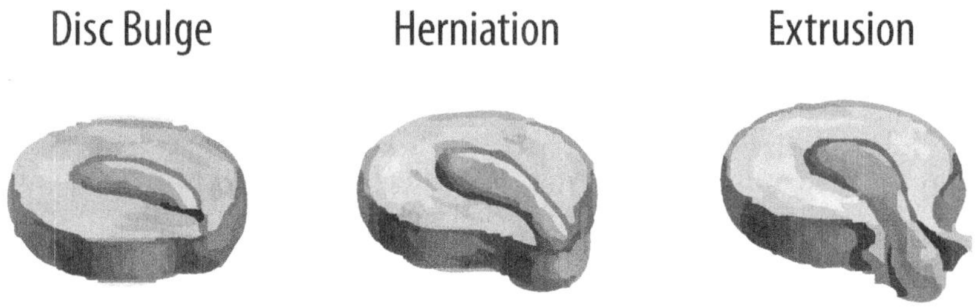

Fig. 16.5: Progression of disc derangement or nuclear displacement.

nucleus has now escaped the confines of the annulus with no way to help it re-enter the broken disc.

The nerve that is being compressed usually becomes inflamed which adds to the painful process. For this reason, many doctors prescribe anti-inflammatory medication that can help reduce the pain. It is not the inflammation however that rapidly reverses when a directional preference is identified and pain rapidly centralizes and abolishes. Rather, it is the compression on the nerve from the herniated disc that can be reversed that enables the pain to reverse as well.

As stated in Chapter 15, as the amount of painful displacement increases, pain spreads farther away from your back or neck, even into the leg or arm (See Figs. 10.3 and 10.4). That displacement also increasingly interferes with the ability of that disc to move freely. Alternatively, if and when the displacement decreases, perhaps as a result of positions and movements identified during the MDT examination, not only does the pain centralize and abolish, but the joint movement improves simultaneously. When the displacement is fully corrected, pain is eliminated and the disc movement returns to normal.

Is your disc pain rapidly reversible?

It is well-documented that a single direction of spinal bending rapidly improves or eliminates full arm or leg pain in 80–90% of recent onset back and neck pain.

One study specifically reports that simply reversing the direction of spine bending actually returns displaced nucleus material to its home or bed in the center of the disc.[62]

So during the MDT examination, centralization of the pain suggests that the disc annulus is still intact and fulfilling its role as a container of the nucleus. This enables the nucleus to be squeezed back to its normal location in the center of the disc. The painful disc has clearly not ruptured. By moving the nucleus away from the back of the disc and away from the nerves that generate pain, the pain rapidly retreats (centralizes) out of the arm or leg, and soon disappears completely.

Do we even need an anatomic diagnosis?

To successfully treat the great majority of back and neck pain, it is enough to simply identify the two mechanical clues of directional preference and pain centralization. They provide sufficient information to effectively treat the problem.[11,13,19,26,28,43,49,63] These two clues indicate two things: 1) your pain source is a derangement, meaning something is out of place, and 2) your problem, the derangement, is *rapidly reversible*, meaning it is reducible and can be quickly put back in place using directional exercises and posture strategies that match your directional preference.

There is fortunately no need to confirm that this is a disc problem. We discussed in Chapter 7 how tricky MRIs and CTs are to interpret in this huge population with back or neck pain. Medications, injections, and surgery are also *unnecessary* in those whose pain can be centralized and eliminated with such simple mechanical exercises and posture changes.

Chapter 17

What if I don't have a *rapidly reversible* problem?

Although most with back or neck pain are fortunate to have a *rapidly reversible* condition, there are some who do not. However, this fairly small subgroup will also benefit from undergoing an MDT examination since the findings of those tests also help guide the next step in care.

Irreversible disc derangement

There are several types of *irreversible* back and neck pain. One is the most extreme stage of the painful disc derangement described in Chapter 16 that has become irreversible. In other words, no directional preference can be found during MDT testing to reduce the displacement and pain.[55,86] The mechanical diagnosis would be an "irreducible derangement." These patients warrant an MRI that routinely confirms the diagnosis of a herniated disc.

With MDT care not helpful, if the severity of the symptoms warrants, one or more epidural steroid injections (ESI) are commonly performed. A steroid is an anti-inflammatory medication placed with a needle in the area of the herniated disc, within what's called the epidural space, where the pain appears to be originating. These injections can reduce or sometimes completely relieve the pain. However, they are not always effective and carry some risk.

When ESIs provide just partial pain relief, a repeat MDT assessment is worthwhile because some painful discs where no directional preference was found before the ESI may now have one.[64] That would be very good news because the newly found directional preference, as always, can provide the means for achieving a successful and full recovery typically by using the indicated directional exercises and posture strategies.

Should ESIs not provide the desired relief, if the individual is sufficiently disabled, and if imaging confirms a clear disc abnormality that explains the pain, *only then* should there be any consideration of disc surgery. Indeed, disc surgery has been shown to be six times more likely in patients whose pain cannot be centralized.[70] It still may be worthwhile waiting for an additional time before deciding on surgery since some will experience a slow shrinking and re-absorption of their displaced disc material. That enables them to improve without surgery, but at a much slower pace.

Non-disc pain

A second type of irreversible back or neck pain does not have the characteristics of a derangement or disc problem on MDT examination. MRI imaging usually reveals no disc abnormality or any other explanation for the pain. Despite no clear spine-related diagnosis, there remain several other possibilities.

Alternative examination tests routinely used by MDT examiners can help determine whether low back pain could be coming from some other joint, like the hip or a sacro-iliac joint,[45,46] which are located on each side of the back of your pelvis. If your pain is determined to be coming from one of those joints, there may be a treatment targeting them that can be helpful.

Treatment options if no directional preference

There remains another very small group who have no directional preference, no other identifiable joint problems, and whose MRI provides no guidance. With no clear diagnosis, several treatment options are commonly utilized. These options are very commonly prescribed treatments for back and neck pain by many clinicians.

► 1—*Back or neck strengthening program.* There is good data showing benefit with this type of care for those with chronic back or neck pain.[48,57] Of course, strengthening is beneficial for everyone, but has been shown to be helpful for those struggling with their recovery from back or neck pain. For those with chronic back or neck pain found to have a directional preference that then fully recover with MDT treatment, there is no evidence of any additional benefit from adding a back or neck strengthening program although this seems like a logical thing to do for someone recovering from a long-term problem.

► 2—*Stabilization exercises.* This very popular treatment attempts to train individuals to function with their spine in "neutral" position. That means intentionally positioning, training, and learning to maintain the painful portion of the spine near the mid-point of its range-of-movement throughout all activities and positions. This approach to care is based on the assumption that minimizing joint movement will both minimize the pain and therefore maximize function.

But recall that it's well established that 80–90% of acute back pain has a directional preference, meaning that the underlying joint problem (disc?) benefits by being moved *fully* to its end-range in a single direction. To instead confine that joint to its mid-range ignores and avoids the very movement that would centralize and abolish the pain and then keep it away. The data showing excellent results using end-range exercises in the majority of back and neck patients are very impressive,[11,13,19,26,28,43,49,63] whereas there are little, if any, published data showing the effectiveness of this stabilization form of care.

Stabilization training, however, has one clear indication. Its primary use should be for those very few whose pain does in fact increase with every direction of end-range testing. In other words, no direction of movement is beneficial. If the severity of pain and disability do not warrant surgery, this very small, but well-defined, group can more comfortably function by training them to function in the middle of their range-of-motion using stabilization exercises.

Unfortunately, many physical therapists prescribe stabilization exercises to treat most or even all back and neck pain, despite the lack of published documentation that it is an effective treatment. Most stabilization advocates have little or no training in the

MDT examination methods and either ignore or are unaware of the evidence that 80–90% of acute and 50% of chronic back pain patients have a directional preference and greatly benefit from moving their spine to its fullest extent in one single direction.

► 3—*Diagnostic injections* are utilized by pain specialists to evaluate other potential sources of pain in individuals with chronic back and neck disorders. Suspected anatomic pain sources are injected to see if either the precise and matching type of pain can be created or aggravated or if a local anesthetic can temporarily stop the pain if placed in the proper location.

► 4—*"Pain management"*: a specialty of care that utilizes special medication combinations (oral and injections) and spinal cord stimulators for chronic and treatment-resistant pain.

► 5—*Multidisciplinary functional restoration program*: assists individuals to become as active and functional as possible without directly addressing the issue of pain. Most studies however report a decrease in pain along with improved function.[33] These were also discussed in Chapter 9.

Most of these treatments are more complex and more expensive and should be discussed with your doctor if your pain is not recovering after having undergone a good MDT evaluation.

Chapter 18

But I've already been to physical therapy and it didn't help.

Physical therapy (PT) is one of the primary professions that provides back and neck pain care. But PT care is highly variable with many different forms of treatment delivered for back and neck pain. So if you've "had physical therapy already," you have likely received just one or two of its many different forms. Reading this book should help clarify whether you've had this MDT form of care or not.

Once again, many have a *rapidly reversible* problem causing their back or neck pain but it has never been discovered because they have never undergone an MDT assessment. Consequently, they frequently undergo other forms of PT treatment, sometimes with little or no progress toward recovery. In many cases, not until the specific directional bending movements needed to reverse the condition are identified and applied will the problem begin to reverse.

Unfortunately, other than MDT care for *rapidly reversible* back and neck pain where a directional preference is found, there is very little evidence that most PT treatments actually improve or speed recoveries. Some treatments, like stabilization exercises (see Chapter 17), appear to offer value for a small subgroup of back or neck pain. The challenge is always to determine the right treatment for the right person.

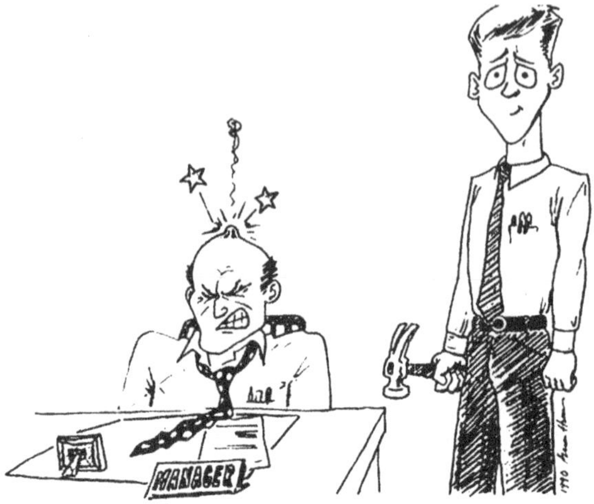

It is often said within the spine care community: "If all you have is a hammer, everything starts looking like a nail." In other words, clinicians look for and find opportunities to use their favorite treatments, usually those in which they are well-trained and therefore enjoy providing. It has often been questioned whether treatment selection might be influenced by what brings the greatest financial reward to the clinician.

Chapter 19

Should I see a chiropractor for my pain?

Individuals struggling with back or neck pain commonly seek pain relief from members of the chiropractic profession. Like all other professions, there is great variation in how chiropractors evaluate and treat their patients.

There is evidence that chiropractic manipulation is beneficial as a short-term treatment for some patients,[6,12,41,78] but many studies report no real benefit compared with other forms of care. But since the risk of making patients worse is low, many chiropractors manipulate nearly everyone in hopes of helping some, but again, often only short-term.

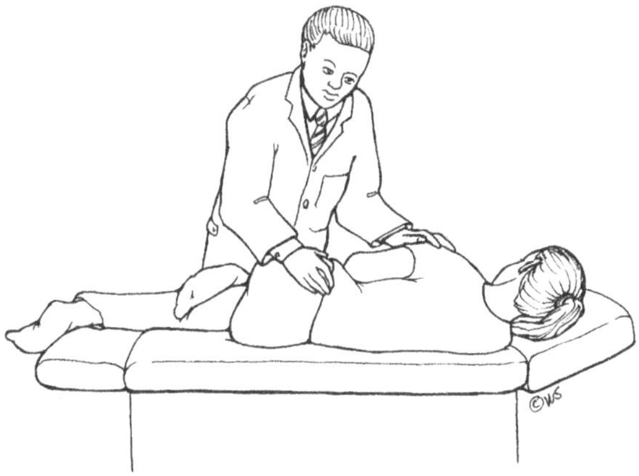

Pain relief from manipulation often lasts for only a few hours, maybe up to a day or two, but then often returns to its prior level. But even short-term relief is attractive when nothing else seems to help. Consequently, many with long-standing neck or back pain pursue these treatments for months, even years, just to receive this short-term relief, over and over, despite no overall improvement in either comfort or activity level.

Many chiropractors use their hands to manipulate the spine

in an effort to correct what they refer to as a spinal misalignment or subluxation. But even chiropractors have difficulty defining these, not to mention trying to *reliably* identify one in a single individual in pain.

That said, many physical therapists also use manipulation in treating back and neck pain and there has been research published on how to identify those patients who might respond to that manipulation.[17] The means of assessing and identifying those patients has been challenged by at least one other study however[35] and there is reason to believe that many who would respond to manipulation also have a *rapidly reversible* problem that could be easily treated without manipulation. This will be discussed later in this chapter.

Patient evaluation

The most troublesome aspect of chiropractic care is the way in which many are taught to evaluate their patients. Many chiropractors routinely use their hands to *feel* the spine and its surrounding tissues in an attempt to determine or learn about the cause of the pain. Feeling with the hands is called "palpation."

Numerous studies have shown the lack of reliability between examiners when using palpation.[66] Again, reliability means that two clinicians examining the same patient can agree on what they feel or palpate. Therefore, without reliability, any conclusions drawn from those tests, including the diagnosis, are essentially useless.

As discussed in Chapter 7, the other troublesome part of some chiropractors' evaluation of back and neck pain patients is their use of x-ray in an effort to identify a misalignment or what is referred to as a "subluxation," meaning something is out of place. However, asymmetries and misalignments are common x-ray findings even in those having no pain.

When found, the chiropractor often portrays to the patient that this is the cause of their pain. This is satisfying information to the explanation-seeking patient. But it ignores the clear lack of evidence that such misalignments are actually painful.

As with palpation, chiropractors are increasingly abandoning the use of these early x-rays in their initial patient evaluations and relying on more reliable forms of examination, such as MDT testing.

Does manipulation have a role within MDT care?

Spinal manipulation applies a mechanical force to the spine in a single direction. Chiropractors, physical therapists, and osteopaths commonly use it. Many who use manipulation typically use it a high percentage of the time with unclear indications for when it is unnecessary.

Patients who experience repeated short-term relief of their back or neck pain from manipulation likely have an unappreciated *rapidly reversible* derangement that is partially reversed by the directional mechanical effect of each manipulation. But the improvement is so often short-term due to the clinicians' lack of understanding of how to maintain the reduction of the derangement necessary to prevent the pain from returning.

That very information is routinely available from the findings of the MDT examination. *Rapidly reversible* derangements not only respond very well to patient-performed directional exercises but, once abolished, those same exercises then usually prevent the return of the pain. Without MDT, these individuals' pain just keeps recurring over and over after temporary relief with manipulation, only to be taken away again and again.

It's quite apparent that any reversible condition could have recovered long, long ago if it had just been evaluated early. Rather than undergoing manipulation again and again and again, it is much better to teach patients effective self-care using directional pain-relieving movements they can perform as needed.

More and more chiropractors are consequently pursuing MDT training in order to identify *rapidly reversible* pain and be able to effectively coach their patients in how to go home, get rid of their own pain and then prevent its return.[22]

An important exception

There is a small but important subgroup of back and neck pain with a directional preference that cannot completely centralize and abolish their pain using end-range exercises. They simply can't produce enough force in their needed direction to fully reduce the displacement. Manipulation can be very helpful by providing the needed additional force at end-range in the needed direction to complete the reduction of the derangement. Manipulation is typically then only needed once or twice since, once the initial reduction is accomplished, the individual can be taught how to keep the pain from returning using directional exercises. This small group is easily identified during the MDT examination.

Dependence vs. independence

If your back or neck problem has a directional preference and you can be taught directional exercises and posture modifications that enable you to eliminate your own problem, your clinician should avoid the use of hands-on interventions like manipulation. Even if manipulation might speed your recovery, it also teaches you a very unfortunate lesson: *dependency upon the clinician.* Whenever your pain returns, you have been taught that manipulation is your answer and you will seek it again, and again, and again. You are far better off learning how to eliminate your own pain and therefore becoming independent of your therapist or chiropractor, able to prevent its return using directional self-treatment strategies.

> "You cannot help men permanently by doing for them what they could or should do for themselves."
>
> —*Abraham Lincoln*

Chapter 20

How do I find an MDT clinician?

It is important for you and your doctor to be able to identify who is and who is not fully trained in MDT methods. Beware that many clinicians claim to know or be trained in these methods when they have had only partial, and sometimes very little, formal training. Some understanding of MDT training is useful in finding someone to help you.

MDT education

The McKenzie Institute International is an educational, non-profit organization that teaches a standardized series of four three- and four-day courses in more than 30 countries. Completion of these four courses qualifies a clinician to take a comprehensive examination to determine if they are able to provide the minimal required elements of MDT care. Those passing this examination are awarded the title of "Credentialed in MDT" and may add "CredMDT" after their name.

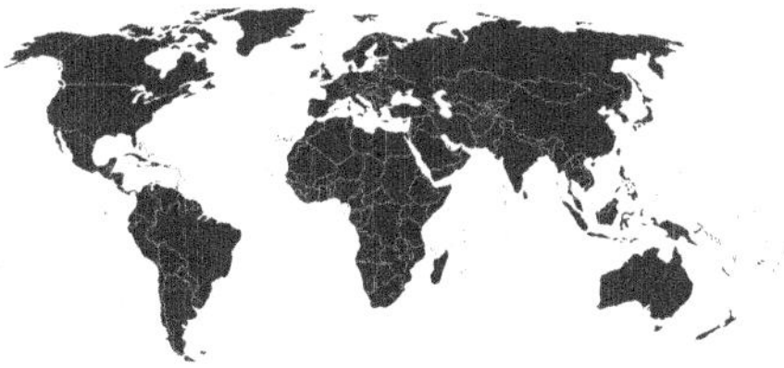

More advanced MDT training is also available consisting of ten weeks of intensive coursework and a nine-week full-time clinical tutorial program. Completion qualifies one to take a second advanced comprehensive examination. Those that pass are granted the title of "Diplomat in MDT" and may add "DipMDT" after their name.

Who is trained in MDT?

The practice of MDT does not belong to any one health care discipline. Ideally, it should be provided by all medical specialties and disciplines for the welfare of everyone who seeks care for their back and neck pain. In reality, most who are formally trained are physical therapists, however a growing number of chiropractors are pursuing training, along with medical doctors, athletic trainers, and exercise physiologists.

Most physicians who want MDT for their patients have chosen not to pursue formal training themselves but instead refer their patients to fully trained clinicians in their communities. Doctors therefore also need to identify the best MDT people available. Fortunately, trained practitioners are available in most communities and that number keeps increasing.

How to find an MDT clinician near you?

For help in finding a trained MDT clinician near you, go to www.mckenziemdt.org. On the left-hand side, a current directory of Credentialed MDT clinicians and Diplomats can be found in your country and state.

If a qualified person is unavailable near you, place phone calls to physical therapy and chiropractic practices near you to inquire who in your community is fully, or nearly fully, trained in MDT. *Be sure to specifically ask who has passed the Credentialing or Diploma examinations or, if no one has, who has taken all, or nearly all, of the four courses offered by the McKenzie Institute.*

Try to be evaluated by the clinician with the most advanced training.

Chapter 21

My doctor says I'm depressed and have fears that are preventing my recovery. Could that be true?

When your pain increases related to your movements and activities, it's natural to become fearful that you are causing further damage. If your pain persists despite pursuing various treatments, your hope of finding a solution may begin to fade. It's easy to begin to conclude you have a "bad" back or neck, which is a depressing thought.

Fear and depression can themselves become obstacles to recovery when they cause you to avoid movement and activity that could otherwise be beneficial. It is commonly believed that being less active is even more detrimental to recovery than pursuing activities, even in pain.

Role of the MDT examination

Despite having pain for many months or years and being understandably depressed and fearful of movement, many still have a *rapidly reversible* condition that has simply never reversed because it has never been discovered and therefore never treated properly (see Chapter 11).

If finally given the opportunity to undergo an MDT evaluation, even in the presence of long-standing pain, fear, and depression, two studies report excellent recoveries using MDT treatment principles that include a significant decrease in fear and depression.[49,85] If a directional preference is identified and specific movements quickly gain control over and eliminate your pain, you quickly realize that you don't have a "bad" back or neck after all and you have nothing further to fear.

Consider this: if you are depressed and fearful of hurting

yourself even more, *what could be more reassuring and uplifting than to discover that you can eliminate your own pain and recover quickly using your own simple movements and positions?* If your pain is *rapidly reversible,* you have an excellent opportunity to fully recover, despite your long-standing pain, fear, and depression.

Alternatively, if you do *not* have a *rapidly reversible* problem, your MDT examiner can quickly determine that as well and promptly steer you toward other care to address your pain, fear, and depression so you may soon become more active (see Chapter 17).

Chapter 22

How to eliminate and prevent most neck and back pain

Self-care options described may not be appropriate for your specific situation. You should talk with your doctor about how the information presented here relates to your specific condition. Your doctor is your final authority in how to address your specific condition.

As discussed in Chapter 15, the mechanical diagnosis for most back and neck pain is a derangement, meaning the underlying condition is likely related to something displaced within a joint that has a directional preference that will reverse or correct it.

By far, the most common preferred direction is "extension," meaning bending the low back or lower neck in a backward direction. The following detail about this form of self-care is offered because of the large percentage of back and neck pain sufferers whose painful condition has an *extension* directional preference. If you were to try these movements and they were not beneficial or in any way aggravated your problem, an assessment with a certified MDT therapist will likely be able to help you find another movement that works better for your pain.

The actual MDT evaluation and treatment of two such patients, one with low back and the other with neck pain, are described in the Appendix. Those cases illustrate the two-part treatment strategy that is critical to providing the most effective result, whether you are attempting to eliminate your current pain or prevent its return and another episode.

Directional exercises

The first strategy of course is exercise, but in the form of specific repeated end-range spine bending movements. An example is described in more detail below. These are always performed in the direction revealed as beneficial during the evaluation.

If trying to eliminate current pain, 8–10 repetitions of that specific movement every two hours should be the goal until the pain is eliminated and stays away. Once pain-free, but wishing to avoid future pain, 8–10 repetitions 1–2 times per day of that same exercise is usually adequate.

Exercises for your lower back

The use of standing backbends (Fig. 22.1), maximally stretching backward with fingers pressed firmly into the small of the back, is simple, convenient, and valuable for treating most low back pain. That backward direction of bending counteracts the aggravating effects of time spent bent forward by decreasing or eliminating the pain. While performing 8–10 repetitions, the ability to bend farther and farther back often increases as well.

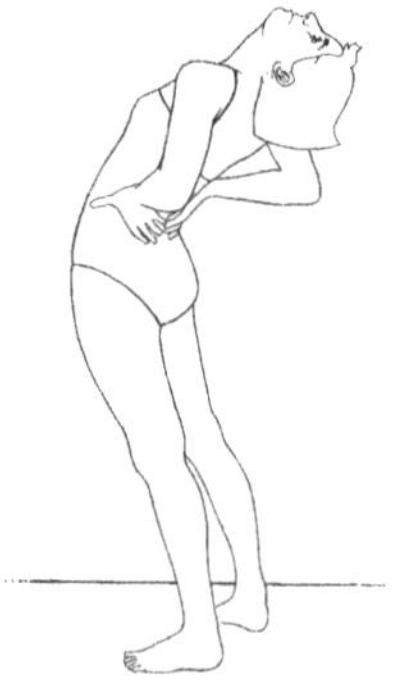

Fig. 22.1: Placing your fingers in the small of your back and bending as far back as possible often reduces, centralizes, abolishes, and prevents lower back pain. Although not always as effective as "press-ups," because it is more convenient, it can be done more frequently, and that has great benefit.

For many, an even more effective way to either eliminate or prevent pain caused by excessive forward bending of the low back is to lie facedown and perform what are commonly referred to as "press-ups" (Fig. 22.2). This exercise is intended to maximize and even increase the depth of the hollow in the low back by pushing the shoulders fully upward with the arms while completely relaxing the mid-section and letting the hips and abdomen sag downward as much as possible.

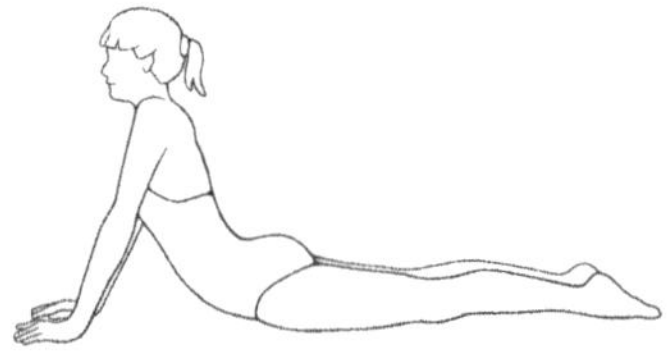

Fig. 22.2: When performed repeatedly to maximize the arch in the lower back, the "press-up" low back exercise often reduces, centralizes, abolishes, and prevents pain coming from a derangement in the lower back.

Performing 8–10 press-ups every two hours, holding the top position for 1–2 seconds before lowering yourself, can be very helpful for most low back pain. If pain interferes at first, lying flat for a bit and then gradually working upward to initially just lean on the elbows can be a very helpful start. As pain and movement improves, progressing to the full press-up should follow.

Exercises for the neck

It is both important and common to be able to eliminate neck pain by counteracting the stresses on the lower neck from the very common and aggravating forward head position (Fig. 22.3). A simple exercise can be very helpful and conveniently done at home or at work.

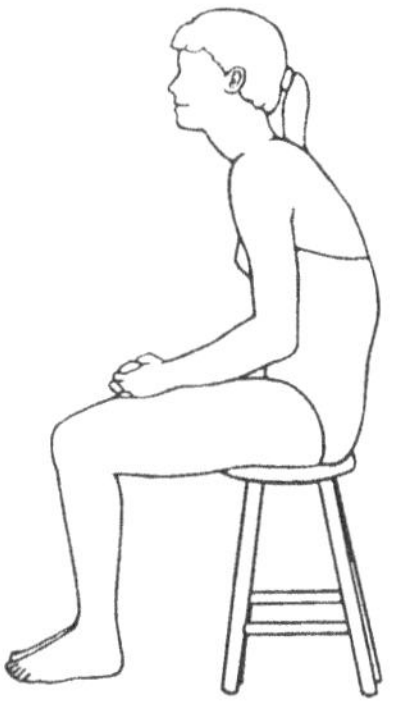

Fig. 22.3: Slouched sitting allows the head to protrude forward and the low back to bend forward for prolonged periods of time. Both the neck and lower back can be aggravated by slouched sitting and correcting this position is usually a key to recovery from and prevention of neck and back pain.

Neck "retractions" or "chin tucks" (Fig. 22.4) are intended to take your head *as far backward as possible while maintaining your face in a forward-looking direction.* By placing your fingers on the front of your chin, you can push your head even farther backward, which is usually beneficial, as long as your pain isn't aggravated when you complete the movement. When done correctly, you will feel a stretch in the back of your neck along with a sense of crowding your throat in front.

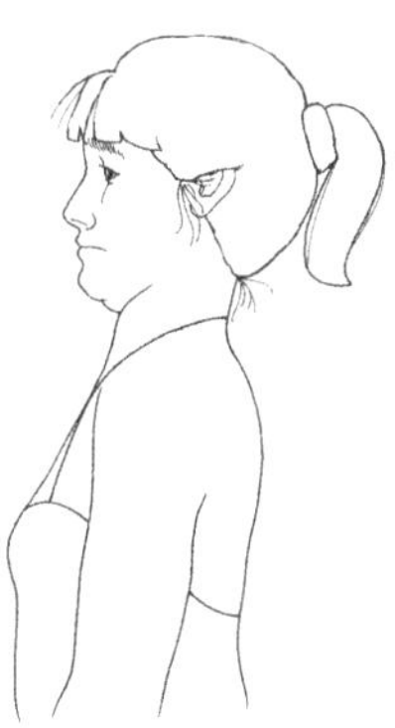

Fig. 22.4: When performed repeatedly to maximize the backward movement of the head, "retraction" often reduces, centralizes, abolishes, and prevents pain coming from a derangement in the lower neck. The effect of the movement can often be increased by placing fingers on the chin to help push the head farther backward, continuing with the face directed straight ahead.

If your pain reduces during the exercise, the head then usually retracts farther and farther backward with each repetition, which allows the exercise to be even more beneficial. This movement should also be done in sets of 8–10 repetitions every two hours until the pain is eliminated.

Once eliminated, sets of this simple exercise performed twice a day will usually help prevent the pain from returning. If pain does return, increasing the frequency again will usually eliminate it fairly quickly.

Insight: to a painful lower neck, retractions are the equivalent of performing backbends for the lower back.

Posture modifications

The second and equally important part of both treatment and prevention is to incorporate proper posture for the low back and neck when not exercising. If directional exercises help reduce the displaced derangement, then time spent between exercise sessions with the spine bent in the opposite direction as part of poor posture can quickly undo much of the good the exercises have achieved. It is critical for both rapid recovery and preventing recurrences to honor the directional preference when not exercising by giving rigorous attention to posture.

Sitting posture: a huge factor in most neck and back pain

The role of posture in the health of our spines cannot be overemphasized. One study reported that simply teaching low back pain patients to sit erectly, with no other treatment, provided a significant reduction and even elimination of their pain compared with those who sat slouched.[87]

The MDT evaluation consistently reveals that the most common thing that creates and aggravates low back pain is time spent with the lower back bent forward, including slouched sitting. It is similar with neck pain. The head protruded forward while sitting, a very common and unfortunate position, requires the lower neck to also be bent forward.

So prolonged and frequent forward bending of both the lower neck and low back occur very commonly with slouched sitting (Fig. 22.3), whether at the computer, in deep soft chairs or sofas while watching TV, sitting up while reading in bed, or when driving your car or truck.

Other forward bending activities: Beside poor posture, there are other forms of forward bending that greatly stress the low back and neck, like vacuuming, working in the garden, or shoveling snow (Fig. 22.5). Lifting, coughing and sneezing also take our backs and necks in that same direction and are frequent contributors to back or neck pain.

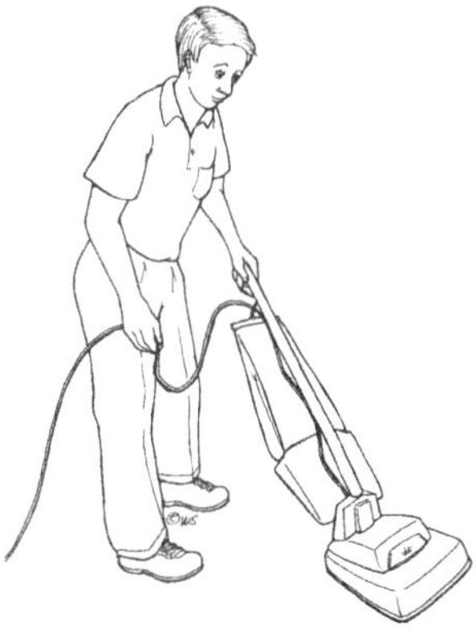

Fig. 22.5: Prolonged time spent with the lower back and neck bent forward with activities like vacuuming, mopping, and garden work often bring on or aggravate persisting back or neck pain.

Sitting erectly: one key to avoiding and eliminating back and neck pain

There are three sitting strategies that are helpful in minimizing these stresses on our backs and necks. The first is to frequently interrupt any prolonged time spent sitting. That's because of the very common habit of sitting with rounding of the entire back while letting the head protrude forward. Getting up to walk provides relief from the stresses on our necks and backs from this aggravating sitting position.

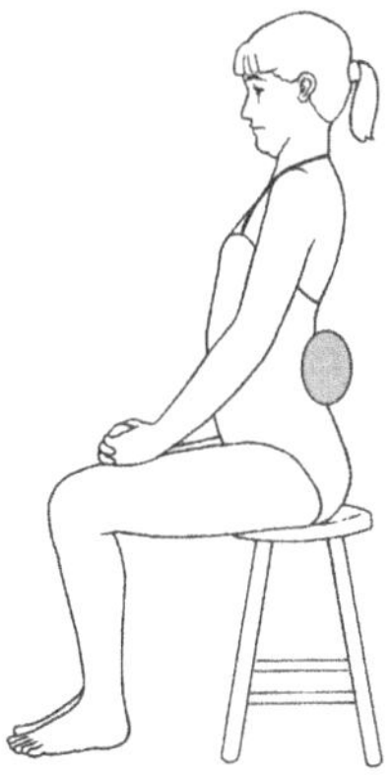

Fig. 22.6: Sitting erectly with your ears directly over the shoulders and with a hollow in the lower back helps decrease and also prevent neck and lower back pain. When in a chair or car seat, adding a support behind the lower back to maintain the same hollow you have when you are walking makes it easier to sit erectly for longer periods of time. Adding that support helps with both neck and low back problems.

Sitting erectly is invaluable. To make that easier, the second strategy is to choose erect and shallower chairs that enable you to rest your feet easily on the floor as you place your buttocks firmly against the lower part of the back of the chair. Avoid deep, low, soft furniture that look very comfortable but require you to slouch.

The third strategy while sitting is to add a lumbar support behind and across the lower back to increase and maintain the same natural hollow while sitting that we have when walking and standing erectly (Fig. 22.6). These can be inexpensively purchased online.

Regarding neck pain, realize that our heads are very heavy so there is much less mechanical stress on the neck if the head is positioned directly over the neck and shoulders, much like placing a golf ball on a golf tee. Ideally our ears should be directly above our shoulders (Fig. 22.6) rather than being positioned forward. The forward or protruded head position requires muscles, ligaments and discs to work hard to keep that heavy head from falling off the front. Those stresses are very similar to forward bending with the lower back for prolonged periods that, in time, becomes painful.

Two excellent and widely read books on these self-care strategies are entitled: *Treat Your Own Back* and *Treat Your Own Neck.*[53,54] Both are written by Robin McKenzie, the renowned back and neck pain expert. They are readily available online and may be very useful in guiding you first in your self-treatment when you are in pain but also for prevention of your pain, once eliminated. The treatment and prevention techniques mentioned above are described in detail in those two books.

What helps prevent back and neck pain?

Someone once said that we prepare for the future by looking at the past. That is certainly true if you have *rapidly reversible* back and neck pain.

Future pain typically has the same directional characteristics as your past pain. It is therefore usually a minor thing if it returns and you promptly return to the exercise and sitting strategies that were so helpful before. So those movements and positions that eliminated your pain in the past are the same ones that will either prevent or quickly eliminate any future pain.

Rapidly reversible pain can and does re-occur if too much of the "wrong" direction of stress is applied that re-creates your derangement. Performing 1–2 sets of your directional exercises each day and remaining diligent about managing your sitting posture are very effective strategies for preventing another derangement episode.

If pain does begin again however, occasionally the exercises that helped you in the past do not seem to work. The mechanics of this new derangement have likely changed just enough from your original ones that a simple modification of your exercise is often all that is needed for you to once again be able gain control over your pain. You should promptly contact your MDT clinician for a quick re-evaluation to sort out what adjustments are needed in your exercises to bring about another rapid recovery.

It is often stated that there is great benefit in staying in good physical condition that includes strengthening, flexibility, and endurance exercise as well as weight loss. These are all valuable for your general health, however they require a great commitment of time and effort compared with the simple prevention methods just described that are far more specific to your particular back or neck problem.

Chapter 23

Summary:

Solving the mystery of your back or neck pain

For all health issues, identifying successful treatment requires sufficient knowledge of the cause of the problem. In the case of most back and neck pain, the cause has been a mystery for a very long time resulting in many different theories and just as many treatments. Experts in a wide range of clinical specialties and disciplines prescribe these treatments and most have failed in research studies to demonstrate effectiveness in helping people recover from their back or neck pain.

Solving the mystery

This mystery has persisted all this time because the relevant information about the cause of back and neck pain is simply unavailable by conventional office examination methods used by most doctors, physical therapists, and chiropractors, as well as the most advanced forms of imaging, like CT and MRI scans.

However, a standardized dynamic examination has been shown in many studies to be capable of reliably revealing excellent clues about the behavior and characteristics of the underlying disorder responsible for most back and neck pain.[15,25,26] Other studies report that these same clues solve a great deal of the mystery for the majority of individuals with back or neck pain by identifying patient-specific treatments that produce rapid, excellent results.[11,13,19,26,28,43,49,63]

This Mechanical Diagnosis & Therapy (MDT) examination dynamically evaluates the underlying pain source using spinal movement and positioning tests that apply different mechanical stresses to it, searching for any test that produces immediate and lasting changes in the intensity and location of the pain. Lasting improvement suggests that something beneficial has been achieved for the pain source.

This improvement is always the result of a single direction of full spinal bending, performed repeatedly. Once this directional preference is identified, rapid and excellent recoveries typically follow using precise directional exercises and posture modifications.[11,13,19,26,28,43,49,63]

> It becomes obvious that your painful condition is being directly treated when both your pain and spinal movement are immediately improved and then remain better.

In 80–90% of acute and in 50% of chronic back and neck pain cases, this MDT examination identifies the presence of two very reliable clues about the cause of your pain: directional preference and pain centralization. If these two clues are found, the underlying condition has the mechanical characteristics of a reducible *derangement.* This means that something is out of place and painful but is capable of being put back into place using a single direction of spinal bending that is usually opposite of the direction of the displacement. That means, in most cases, the underlying cause is mechanical as well as *rapidly reversible.*

There is good evidence that this derangement type of pain may be caused by displacement of the nucleus of an intervertebral disc.[62] Fortunately, it is not necessary to prove or confirm this in order for most individuals to effectively treat themselves and recover. It is adequate to simply determine that your condition is *rapidly reversible* and to learn what directional movements and positions relieve and eliminate the pain and then keep it away.

It is important that clinicians who perform this MDT examination be well trained in order to avoid missing many who have this *rapidly reversible* problem. When derangements remain undiscovered and therefore untreated, they often progress to develop either chronic problems or require surgery.

> No matter how severe your pain is, how long you've had it, how many episodes you've had, how far down your arm or leg it has spread, or how many prior unsuccessful treatments you have tried, your painful back or neck condition could still have a directional preference and be rapidly reversible.

Of course there are some whose pain source does not have an identifiable directional preference. However, other MDT examination findings often place them into other small subgroups that help guide the selection of effective treatments.

Bad news . . .

More than 80% of adults experience low back or neck pain at some point. The United States spends $80–100 *billion* each year on those disabled by and seeking treatment for these conditions, largely because the cause of most back and neck pain remains a mystery to most clinicians.

Good news . . .

Solving a very large part of that mystery is a major breakthrough. That the great majority of back or neck pain is caused by a *rapidly reversible* derangement is excellent news for those struggling with it, and certainly for those who pay for all the unnecessary care, including most employers, and for all those clinicians whose priority is to find simple, safe, reliable, and rapid solutions for their patients with back and neck pain.

A detailed review of the scientific evidence that supports the content of this book is presented in another Self-Care First publication (www.selfcarefirst.com) entitled *Rapidly Reversible Low Back Pain: An Evidence-based Pathway to Widespread Recoveries and Cost-Savings.*

Appendix

Case of rapidly reversible chronic low back and left leg pain

Clare was 52 years old when she developed a sore back after moving some furniture. When her pain worsened, she saw her family doctor who sent her to physical therapy, but that was not all that helpful. During treatment, her pain even began to spread down her left leg. Her doctor and therapist nevertheless felt she should continue physical therapy and was also given anti-inflammatory medications.

With more and more flare-ups, she was referred to an orthopedic specialist. An MRI was ordered but she was told it didn't show very much. She was told to continue physical therapy even though it didn't seem to be helping her.

She saw a second orthopedic specialist who also felt it would simply take more time and she needed to become more fit. Physical therapy was continued but now her left leg pain had become constant and so painful she was unable to continue working.

A second MRI higher up in her back showed some herniated discs in her thoracic (chest portion) spine but those were not considered responsible for her pain.

One of her orthopedic surgeons discussed the option of surgery and referred her to a neurosurgeon who found nothing to operate on and labeled her as having "chronic pain."

She was sent to a pain specialist who told her she would have to learn how to live with her pain and manage it with drugs. She was evaluated by a "specialty team" consisting of an occupational medicine physician, physical therapist, and psychologist. They developed a plan that would include an intense rehabilitation program.

She had now been in pain for two years. It had become

constant with shooting pain down her left leg and she was too painful to work.

Through another contact, she was finally given the opportunity to see a physical therapist well-trained in Mechanical Diagnosis & Therapy (MDT).

The therapist learned that prolonged sitting would consistently bring on or worsen her leg pain and observed that she sat very slouched. By having her sit very erectly, Clare reported that the intensity of her leg pain promptly decreased. When she repeatedly extended her lower back (bent backward), her leg pain decreased more and more until it disappeared. Slouched sitting would bring the pain back again but she found she could decrease and eliminate her leg pain with backward bending while standing or sitting but was especially effective when lying facedown performing a series of press-ups (Fig. 22.2).

The therapist explained that her pain had clearly "centralized" (come out of her leg) with low back extension test movements and this was a very good sign. She likely had a bulging disc that was irritating a nerve causing the pain, numbness and tingling in her leg. The longer she sits slouched, the more it bulges and the pain increases. But extension (backbending) likely decreases that bulge by putting the displaced disc material back in its place that then takes the pressure off the nerve.

It was important to find out whether she would be able to stop her pain and keep it from returning using these extension exercises and very erect sitting posture. Could she now prevent the leg pain from returning and eliminate whatever low back pain was still present?

She was given a lumbar roll to place behind her lower back whenever sitting (Fig. 22.6) to help her avoid the slouch and she was to perform 10–12 press-ups (Fig. 22.2) 5–6 times per day for the next several days. She needed to be seen for another 2–3 visits to be sure that this was working.

With considerable hope that something useful had been found, Clare began to work diligently on her sitting posture and performed her exercises as instructed. By doing so, when she returned two days later, she reported she was able to stop her leg pain herself and even keep it from returning.

She was encouraged to keep up the same self-care efforts. She soon found herself pain-free and off all medications. She was also able to become much more active and soon was able to return to work.

In hindsight, despite two years of worsening pain, seeing numerous physicians, therapists, and a psychologist, despite having had two MRIs, lots of medications, and nearly two years of physical therapy, it is clear that Clare had a *rapidly reversible* problem all that time that simply had never been evaluated adequately or discovered. Unfortunately, none of her physicians or physical therapists ever provided the MDT evaluation nor sent her to someone who could.

Clare had been unnecessarily doomed by all her care givers to a life of "chronic pain" while her true problem, when finally fully evaluated using MDT principles, was actually a *rapidly reversible* derangement that she was able to easily correct herself and then able to maintain that correction and get back to work and her life.

Case of rapidly reversible chronic neck whiplash injury with left arm pain

Peter is a 38-year-old adventure guide and instructor who was on his honeymoon when the car he was driving was hit from behind while stopped. He passed out at the scene and was taken by ambulance to the hospital where no severe injuries were identified. He was discharged, given Tylenol, and told to see his doctor when he returned home.

Severe headaches soon started that kept him from sleeping at night as well as pain and numbness progressing down his left arm to his hand. His physician at home sent him to physical therapy that he continued for 18 months.

His pain forced him to stop working because he couldn't rotate his head when kayaking or look upward when leading rock-climbing groups.

A neck MRI showed bulging/prolapsed discs at his C5–6 and C6–7 levels that were pressing against his nerve causing the pain and tingling in his left arm.

He was referred to a neurosurgeon who offered him surgery to relieve the pressure on the nerve. He was told there was a 50% chance of improvement, 40% chance of being the same, and a 10% chance of worsening as a result of the surgery. Because he didn't like those odds, he decided against surgery.

He was finally given the opportunity to be examined by a physical therapist with extensive training in Mechanical Diagnosis & Therapy (MDT). At that time, he reported he had improved only 10% over his 18 months of physical therapy. He had pain, numbness and tingling into his left palm and fingers as well as tension and tightness in his neck and aching in his left arm. He did report some improvement in those symptoms four months earlier when he changed his job and stopped climbing and kayaking.

Attempts to bend his neck in any direction seemed to increase his neck and arm pain, including bending his head and neck backward. But a special variation of neck extension (bending the neck backward) noticeably decreased the arm and hand tingling that then didn't return, which he stated was a "huge difference" from his last 18 months. With more neck extension movements, his hand and arm symptoms improved substantially and remained better, which greatly impressed Peter.

The therapist told Peter that something was pressing on the nerve and they were perhaps learning that this "something" might be able to be withdrawn from the nerve so his pain and tingling would go away.

He was instructed to perform 10–12 repetitions of the cervical extension exercises 5–6 times/day. He was shown how to perform them standing, sitting and lying down. He was shown how his forward head position when sitting aggravated his condition and was given a lumbar roll to use behind his lower back, especially in the car, to enable him to sit more erectly with his head positioned much better to keep from aggravating his condition while sitting (Fig. 22.6).

Using this self-care strategy, the tingling in his arm and hand disappeared almost immediately despite having been present for 18 months. His headache, neck and arm pain progressively decreased over the next four weeks to where he no longer had any pain. He reported three months later that he was pain-free as long as he did his exercises. He admitted to only doing them 1–2 times per day and if he stopped those exercises for more than two days, his headaches would return very slightly which reminded him to return to his exercises.

He had been able to return to his work and had even taken up snowboarding as a new sport that he could now include in his work.

Like Clare, Peter had an undiscovered *rapidly reversible* problem all this time. Like so many with motor vehicle whiplash injuries, his neck and arm pain didn't begin until many days after his accident. He then underwent 18 months of useless physical therapy and almost accepted an unnecessary surgical procedure because neither he nor his physicians knew his underlying problem was actually *rapidly reversible* the whole time. Fortunately, Peter finally found someone trained to evaluate and treat him using MDT principles of care.

These two cases were selected for presentation because readers can actually observe these two individuals undergoing their MDT evaluation and treatment on a DVD that can be purchased at http://www.optp.com/A-Day-with-McKenzie-DVD_914DVD.aspx. The therapist on the DVD who assessed Clare and Peter is Robin McKenzie, who developed the MDT method of care (see Chapter 12).

Glossary of back and neck pain terms

Acute: having developed recently, often defined as starting within 4 weeks.

Annulus fibrosis: the intervertebral disc's outer shell or envelope.

CAT (computer-axial tomography) or CT scan: these mean the same thing: an imaging test that uses radiation to show three-dimensional detail about the bones and joints of the spine with minimal detail regarding soft tissues like ligaments, discs and muscles.

Centralization: the retreat of referred or radiating pain back toward the spine or center of the human body. Movements that cause such a retreat are said to "centralize" the pain.

Chronic: long standing, often defined as lasting at least 12 weeks.

Degenerative arthritis: also referred to as osteoarthritis in non-spine joints or as degenerative disc disease (DDD) in the spine. It is a wear-and-tear form of joint degeneration, sometimes resulting from a prior trauma to the joint. X-rays of many non-painful joints show signs of this form of degeneration. Pain can result if the degeneration is severe enough but that is difficult to determine from the x-ray appearance of the joint, especially with DDD of the spine.

Derangement: the displacement of tissue with a joint that is painful and interferes with normal movement of the joint. Certain postures and movements worsen the symptoms while others both improve them and restore normal movement to the joint.

Directional preference: a single direction of spinal bending, typically performed repeatedly to the available extreme position (to end-range), that causes symptoms to centralize, diminish, or abolish.

Discs: the soft, rubber-like structures found between the vertebrae of the spine; comprised of an outer shell or envelope (the annulus fibrosis) and an inner gel (the nucleus pulposus). Discs serve as shock absorbers and joints between the vertebrae and change their shape (wedge in various directions) in order for the spine to bend.

Epidural steroid injection (ESI): an injection of cortisone into the space within the spinal column where the suspected pain-producing disc and nerve are located. The purpose is to have the cortisone reduce or eliminate any inflammation that might be present as part of the pain production. These injections are often carried out in a series of three.

Extension: when applied to the spine, this is any form of backward-directed bending.

Facet joint: one of a matched pair of small joints, located on the left and right side of each level of the spine, that, together with the intervertebral disc, comprise the three-joints that control and allow motion between adjacent vertebrae.

Flexion: when applied to the spine, this is any form of forward-directed bending, including sitting slouched, bringing knees to the chest, forward leaning or bending, or lifting.

Herniated disc (also protruding, bulging, ballooning, or slipped disc): a condition in which a tear in the outer, fibrous envelope (the annulus) of an intervertebral disc allows the soft, central portion (the nucleus) to bulge outward. It may or may not be a source of pain, but when it is, the pain often extends down the arm (neck herniation) or leg (low back herniation) if a nerve outside the disc is irritated by the herniation. When the leg pain extends below the knee, it is often referred to as sciatica.

Joint: where one bone meets or connects with another using soft tissue (ligaments, joint capsule, muscles) to support and allow controlled movement between the two bones.

Ligament: a strong band of tissue that spans a joint, restricting joint movement in certain directions while allowing it in others.

Mechanical Diagnosis & Therapy: a method of evaluation and non-surgical treatment of painful spine and extremity joint disorders. The evaluation is based on symptom response to test movements that provide a reliable means of classifying each disorder a valid subgroup for which effective subgroup-specific treatment can usually be identified. Treatment typically consists of a single specific exercise performed by the person in pain (active treatment), along with posture modifications, vs. treatment provided to them by someone else (passive treatment).

MRI (Magnetic Resonance Imaging): an imaging test that shows bones, joints, ligaments discs, and nerves in the spine. MRI stands for "magnetic resonance imaging."

Narcotic: a morphine-class drug for pain relief; example Oxycodone (Percocet).

Non-steroidal anti-inflammatory drug (NSAID): any of several medicines with two properties: inflammation and pain reduction.

Nucleus pulposus: the intervertebral disc's inner jell that moves and changes its shape as the spine is bent in various directions.

Rapidly reversible pain: pain that can be rapidly centralized, reduced or eliminated, almost always as a result of a single direction of end-range spinal bending tests, and can also then be re-produced as a result of prolonged or repeated bending of the spine, usually in the opposite direction of what improves or eliminates the pain.

Sacroiliac joint: a long, irregular, vertically-oriented joint that joins the sacrum, the lowest part of our spine just above our tailbone, with the right and left ilia. Each ilium includes most of the left or right half of the pelvis, including the iliac crests, the ridges of bone felt running around each side at the waistline. The left and right sacroiliac joints have very little movement and can be a cause of pain.

Sciatica: pain extending from the lower back or buttock down the back of the leg past the knee, sometimes spreading into the ankle or foot; usually caused by pressure on the sciatic nerve which runs from the lower back down the back of the thigh to the calf.

Vertebrae: bones that make up the spine from the top of the neck to the tailbone. Vertebrae surround and protect the spinal cord. Vertebra means one of these bones while vertebrae mean two or more of them.

X-ray: an imaging test that uses radiation to visualize primarily the bones of the body.

References

1. Adams M, Hutton W. Gradual disc prolapse. *Spine*. 1985;10:524–31.
2. Adams MA, May S, Freeman BJ, Morrison HP, Dolan P. Effects of backward bending on lumbar intervertebral discs. Relevance to physical therapy treatments for low back pain. *Spine*. 2000;25(4):431–7; discussion 8.
3. Aina S, May S, Clare H. The centralization phenomenon of spinal symptoms—a systematic review. *Manual Therapy*. 2004;9:134–43.
4. Andersson G. Epidemiologic features of chronic low back pain. *Lancet*. 1999;354:581–5.
5. Ash L, Modic M, Obuchowski N, Ross J, Brant-Zawadzki M, Grooff P. Effects of diagnostic information, per se, on patient outcomes in acute radiculopathy and low back pain. *American Journal of Neuroradiology*. 2008;29:109–3.
6. Assendelft W, Morton S, Yu E, Suttorp M, Shekelle P. Spinal manipulative therapy for low back pain. a meta-analysis of effectiveness relative to other therapies. *Annals of Internal Medicine*. 2003;138:871–81.
7. Atlas SJ, Deyo RA. Evaluating and managing acute low back pain in the primary care setting. *J Gen Intern Med*. 2001;16(2):120–31.
8. Bach S, Holten K. Guideline update: What's the best approach to acute low back pain? *Journal of Family Practice*. 2009;58:E1–3.
9. Boden S, Davis D, Dina T. Abnormal magnetic-resonance scans of the lumbar spine in asymptomatic subjects: a prospective investigation. *Journal of Bone and Joint Surgery*. 1990;72:403–8.
10. Boos N, Dreier D, Hilfiker E, Schade V, Kreis R, Hora J, et al. Tissue characterization of symptomatic and asymptomatic disc herniations by quantitative magnetic resonance imaging. *Journal of Orthopaedic Research*. 1997;15(1):141–9.
11. Brennan G, Fritz J, Hunter S, Thackeray A, Delitto A, Erhard R. Identifying subgroups of patients with acute/subacute "nonspecific" low back pain. Results of a randomized clinical trial. *Spine*. 2006;31:623–31.
12. Bronfort G, Haas M, Evans R, Bouter L. Efficacy of spinal manipulation and mobilization for low back pain and neck pain: a systematic review and best evidence synthesis. *The Spine Journal*. 2004;4:335–56.
13. Browder D, Childs J, Cleland J, Fritz J. Effectiveness of an extension-oriented treatment approach in a subgroup of patients with low back pain: a randomized clinical trial. *Physical Therapy*. 2007;87(12):1–11.
14. Bybee R, Olsen D, Cantu-Boncser G, Allen H, Byars A. Centralization of symptoms and lumbar range of motion in patients with low back pain. *Physiotherapy Theory and Practice*. 2009;25:257–67.
15. Cabana M, Rand C, Powe N, Wu A, Wilson M, Abboud P, et al. Why don't physicians follow clinical practice guidelines? a framework for improvement. *Journal of the American Medical Association*. 1999;282.
16. Cherkin D, Deyo R, Wheeler K, Ciol M. Physician variation in diagnostic testing for low back pain: who you see is what you get. *Arthritis and Rheumatism*. 1994;37(1):15–22.
17. Childs J, Fritz J, Flynn T, Irrgang J, Johnson K, Majkowski G, et al. A clinical prediction rule to identify patients with low back pain most likely to benefit from spinal manipulation: a validation study. *Annals of Internal Medicine*. 2004;141:920–8.
18. Chorti A, Chortis A, Strimpakos N, McCarthy C, Lamb S. The prognostic value of symptom responses in the conservative management of spinal pain: a systematic review. *Spine*. 2009;34:2686–99.
19. Clare H. Missing evidence. *British Medical Journal*. 2007;332:0–a.
20. Croft P, Joseph S, Cosgrove S, Jordan L, Papageorgiou A, Pope D, et al. Low back pain in the community and in hospitals. *A Report to the Clinical Standards Advisory Group of the Department of Health*. Manchester, UK: The Arthritis and Rheumatism Council, Epidemiology Research Unit And The Rheumatic Diseases Center, University of Manchester, February 1994.

21. Croft P, Macfarlane G, Papageorgiou A, Thomas E, Silman A. Outcome of low back pain in general practice: a prospective study. *British Medical Journal.* 1998;316:1356–9.
22. DeFoyd W. Chiropractic treatment. In: Deregery J, Anderson J, editors. *Low back pain: an evidence-based, biopsychosocial model for clinical management.* Beverly Farms, MA: OEM Press; 2002. p. 280.
23. Deyo R, Diehl A. Patient satisfaction with medical care for low-back pain. *Spine.* 1986;11:28–30.
24. Deyo R, Diehl A, Rosenthal M. How many days of bed rest for acute low back pain? A randomized clinical trial. *NEJM.* 1986;315:1064–70.
25. Donelson R. Evidence-based low back care? *British Medical Journal.* 2007;332(7555):0–a.
26. Donelson R. Letter to the Editor: The reliability of centralized pain response. *Arch Phys Med Rehab.* 2000;81:999–1000.
27. Donelson R. *Rapidly reversible low back pain: an evidence-based pathway to widespread recoveries and savings.* Hanover, NH: SelfCare First, LLC; 2007.
28. Donelson R, Aprill C, Medcalf R, Grant W. A prospective study of centralization of lumbar and referred pain: A predictor of symptomatic discs and anular competence. *Spine.* 1997;22(10):1115–22.
29. Donelson R, Grant W, Kamps C, Medcalf R. Pain response to repeated end-range sagittal spinal motion: a prospective, randomized, multi-centered trial. *Spine.* 1991;16(6S):206–12.
30. Donelson R, McIntosh G, Hall H, editors. Should we rethink the natural history of low back pain? The International Forum for Primary Care Research in Low Back Pain; 2009 June 2009; Boston, MA, USA.
31. Donelson R, Silva G, Murphy K. The centralization phenomenon: its usefulness in evaluating and treating referred pain. *Spine.* 1990;15(3):211–13.
32. Fennell A, Jones A, Hukins D. Migration of the nucleus pulposus within the intervertebral disc during flexion and extension of the spine. *Spine.* 1996;21:2753–7.
33. Guzmán J, Esmail R, Karjalainen K, Malmivaara A, Irvin E, Bombardier C. Multidisciplinary rehabilitation for chronic low back pain: systematic review. *British Medical Journal.* 2001;322:1511–6.
34. Hagan K, Hilde G, Jamtvedt G, Winnem M. The updated Cochrane review of bed rest for low back pain and sciatica. *Spine.* 2005;30(5):542–6.
35. Hancock M, Maher C, Latimer J, Herbert R, McAuley J. Independent evaluation of a clinical prediction rule for spinal manipulative therapy: a randomised controlled trial. *Eur Spine J.* 2008;17:936–43.
36. Hart G, Deyo R, Cherkin D. Physicians office visits for low back pain: frequency, clinical evaluation, and treatment patterns from a national survey. *Spine.* 1995;10(1):1–9.
37. Henschke N, Maher C, Refshauge K, Herbert R, Cumming R, Bleasel J, et al. Prevalence of and screening for serious spinal pathology in patients presenting to primary care settings with acute low back pain. *Arthritis & Rheumatism.* 2009;60(10):3072–80.
38. Hill J, Dunn K, Lewis M, Mullis R, CJ M, Foster N, et al. A primary care back pain screening tool: identifying patient subgroups for initial treatment. *Arthritis & Rheumatism* (Arthritis Care & Research). 2008;59:632–41.
39. Jensen M, Brant-Zawadski M, N O, Modic M, Malkasian D, Ross J. Magnetic resonance imaging of the lumbar spine in people without back pain. *NEJM.* 1994;331:69–73.
40. Karas R, McIntosh G, Hall H, Wilson L, Melles T. The relationship between non-organic signs and centralization of symptoms in the prediction of return to work for patients with low back pain. *Physical Therapy.* 1997;77(4):354–60.
41. Koes B, Assendelft W, Van der Heijden G, Bouter L. Spinal manipulation for low back pain. *Spine.* 1996;24:2860–71.
42. Koes B, van Tulder M, Ostelo R, Burton A, Waddell G. Clinical guidelines for the management of low back pain in primary care. An international comparison. *Spine.* 2001;26:2504–14.
43. Kopp J, Alexander A, Turocy R, Levrini M, Lichtman D. The use of lumbar extension in the evaluation and treatment of patients with acute herniated nucleus pulposus, a preliminary report. *Clinical Orthopedics.* 1986;202:211–8.

44. Kuslich S, Ulstrom C. The tissue origin of low back pain and sciatica: a report of pain response to tissue stimulation during operations on the lumbar spine using local anesthesia. *Ortho Clin N Amer.* 1991;22(2):181–7.
45. Laslett M. Evidence-based diagnosis and treatment of the painful sacroiliac joint. *Journal of Manual and Manipulative Therapy.* 2008;16:142–52.
46. Laslett M, Aprill C, McDonald B, Young S. Diagnosis of sacroiliac joint pain: validity of individual provocation tests and composites of tests. *Manual Therapy.* 2005;10:207–18.
47. Laslett M, Öberg B, Aprill C, McDonald B. Centralization as a predictor of provocation discography results in chronic low back pain, and the influence of disability and distress on diagnostic power. *The Spine Journal.* 2005;5:370–80.
48. Leggett S, Mooney V, Matheson L, Nelson B, Dreisinger T, Van Zytveld J, et al. Restorative exercise for clinical low back pain: a prospective two-center study with 1-year follow-up. *Spine.* 1999;24:889.
49. Long A, Donelson R, Fung T. Does it matter which exercise? A randomized controlled trial of exercise for low back pain. *Spine.* 2004;29(23):2593–602.
50. Luo X, Pietrobon R, Sun S, Liu B, Hey L. Estimates and patterns of direct health care expenditures among individuals with back pain in the United States. *Spine.* 2004;29:79–86.
51. Martin B, Deyo R, Mirza S, Turner J, Comstock B, Hollingworth W, et al. Expenditures and health status among adults with back and neck problems. *JAMA.* 2008;299(6):656–64.
52. McKenzie R. *The lumbar spine: mechanical diagnosis and therapy.* Waikanae, New Zealand: Spinal Publications; 1981.
53. McKenzie R. *Treat your own back.* Waikanae, New Zealand: Spinal Publications; 1997.
54. McKenzie R. *Treat your own neck.* Waikanae, New Zealand: Spinal Publications; 1997.
55. McKenzie R, May S. *Mechanical Diagnosis and Therapy.* Second ed. Waikanae, New Zealand: Spinal Publications New Zealand Ltd.; 2003.
56. Mooney V, Robertson J. The facet syndrome. *Clinical Orthopedics.* 1976;115:149–55.
57. Nelson B, Carpenter D, Dreisinger T, Mitchel M, Wegner JA. Can spinal surgery be prevented by aggressive strengthening exercises? A prospective study of cervical and lumbar patients. *Archives of Physical Medicine & Rehabilitation.* 1999;80:20–5.
58. O'Neill C, Kurgansky M, Derby R, Ryan D. Disc stimulation and patterns of referred pain. Spine. 2002;27(24):2776–81.
59. Pengel L, Herbert R, Maher C, Refshauge K. Acute low back pain: systematic review of its prognosis. *British Medical Journal.* 2003;327:323–8.
60. Rasmussen C, Nielsen G, Hansen V, Jensen O, Schioettz-Christensen B. Rates of lumbar disc surgery before and after implementation of multidisciplinary nonsurgical spine clinics. *Spine.* 2005;30:2469–73.
61. Rossignol M, Arsenault B, Dionne C, Poitras S, Tousignant M, Truchon M, et al. Clinic on low-back pain in interdisciplinary practice (CLIP) guidelines. Montréal: Direction de santé publique, Agence de la santé et des services sociaux de Montréal. 2007.
62. Scannell J, McGill S. Disc prolapse: evidence of reversal with repeated extension. *Spine.* 2009;34:344–50.
63. Schenk R, Jazefczyk C, Kopf A. A randomized trial comparing interventions in patients with lumbar posterior derangement. *J Manip Phys'l Ther.* 2003;11(2):95–102.
64. Schepers M, van Helvoirt H, editors. Identification and management of irreducible derangements. 11th International Conference in Mechanical Diagnosis and Therapy; 2009 August 30, 2009; Rio de Janeiro, Brazil.
65. Schnebel B, Simmons J, Chowning J, Davidson R. A digitizing technique for the study of movement of intradiscal dye in response to flexion and extension of the lumbar spine. *Spine.* 1988;13(3):309–12.
66. Seffinger M, Majm W, Mkishra S, Adams A, Dickerson V, Murphy L, et al. Reliability of spinal palpation for diagnosis of back and neck pain. A systematic review of the literature. *Spine.* 2004;29:E413–25.
67. Seroussi R, Krag M, Muller D, al e. Internal deformations of intact and enucleated human lumbar discs subjected to compression, flexion, and extension loads. *Journal of Orthopedic Research.* 1989;7(1):122–30.
68. Shepherd J. In vitro study of segmental motion in the lumbar spine. *Journal of Bone and Joint Surgery.* 1995;77B:S2:161.

69. Sizer Jr P, Brismée J, Cook C. Medical screening for red flags in the diagnosis and management of musculoskeletal spine pain. *Pain Practice*. 2007;7:53–71.
70. Skytte L, May S, Petersen P. Centralization—its prognostic value in patients with referred symptoms and sciatica. *Spine*. 2005;30:E(293–9).
71. Smith-Bindman R, Lipson J, Marcus R, al. e. Radiation dose associated with common computed tomography examinations and the associated lifetime attributable risk of cancer. Arch Intern Med 2009;169:2078–2086. Arch Intern Med. 2009(169):2078–86.
72. Smyth M, Wright V. Sciatica and the Intervertebral Disc. *Journal of Bone and Joint Surgery*. 1958;40A:1410.
73. Spitzer W, LeBlanc F, Dupuis M. Scientific approach to the assessment and management of activity-related spinal disorders (The Quebec Task Force). *Spine*. 1987;12(7S):S16–21.
74. Sufka A, Hauger B, Trenary M, Hagan A, Lozon R, Martens B. Centralization of low back pain and perceived functional outcome. *Journal of Orthopedics and Sports Physical Therapy*. 1998;27(3):205–12.
75. Thelander U, Fagerlud M, Friberg S, larsson S. Describing the size of lumbar disc herniations using computed tomography. A comparison of different size index calculations and their relation to sciatica. *Spine*. 1994;19:1979–84.
76. Udermann B, Spratt K, Donelson R, Mayer J, Graves J, Tillotson J. Can a patient educational book change behavior and reduce pain in chronic low back pain patients? *The Spine Journal*. 2004;4:425–35.
77. van Tulder M, Becker A, Bekkering T, Breen A, Gil de Real T, Hutchinson A, et al. European guidelines for the management of acute non-specific low back pain in primary care. [http://www.backpaineurope.org/web/html/evidence.html] 2004 [updated November 10–13, 2004].
78. van Tulder M, Koes B, Bouter L. Conservative treatment of acute and chronic nonspecific low back pain: a systematic review of randomized controlled trials of the most common interventions. *Spine*. 1997;22:2128–56.
79. Verbeek JM, Sengers M, Riemens L, Haafkens J. Patient expectations of treatment for back pain: a systematic review of qualitative and quantitative studies. *Spine*. 2004;29:2309–18.
80. Videman T, Nurminen M. The occurrence of annular tears and their relation to lifetime back pain history: a cadaveric study using barium sulfate discography. *Spine*. 2004;29:2668–76.
81. Von Korff M. Studying the natural history of back pain. *Spine*. 1994;19(18 Suppl):2041S–6S.
82. Von Korff M, Saunders K. The course of back pain in primary care. *Spine*. 1996;21:2833–7.
83. Wasiak R, Kim J, Pransky G. Work disability and costs caused by recurrence of low back pain: longer and more costly than in first episodes. Spine. 2006;31:219–25.
84. Waxman R, Tennant A, Helliwell P. A prospective follow-up study of low back pain in the community. *Spine*. 2000;25(16):2085–90.
85. Werneke M, Hart DL, Cook D. A descriptive study of the centralization phenomenon. A prospective analysis. Spine. 1999;24(7):676–83.
86. Wetzel T, Donelson R. The role of repeated end-range/pain response assessment in the management of symptomatic lumbar discs. The Spine Journal. 2003;3:146–54.
87. Williams M, Hawley J, McKenzie R, Van Wijmen P. A comparison of the effects of two sitting postures on back and referred pain. *Spine*. 1991;16(10):1185–91.
88. Witt I, Vestergaard A, Rosenklint A. A comparative analysis of x-ray findings of lumbar spine in patients with and without lumbar pain. *Spine*. 1984;9:298–300.
89. Wyke B. Neurological aspects of low back pain. In: Jayson J, editor. *The lumbar spine and back pain*. New York: Grune and Stratton; 1976.

Index

Made in the USA
Monee, IL
08 November 2026

67380481R00069